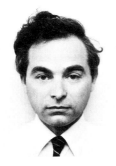

Dr Bernard Valman is a Consultant Pediatrician at Northwick Park Hospital and the Medical Research Council Clinical Research Center in North London. Babies and children of all ages with acute or chronic problems are seen in the pediatric unit, which also includes a section for the intensive care of the newborn.

He is the Secretary of the Pediatric Committee of the Royal College of Physicians and member of the Child Health Computer Committee of the Department of Health. He has written several research articles and books.

He has directed two full length films on child health and also made videotapes for family doctors.

He has also held posts in the Hospital for Sick Children, Great Ormond Street, and the Queen Elizabeth Hospital for Children in London.

His hobbies are gardening and medical writing. He is married and has two children.

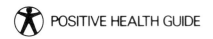
POSITIVE HEALTH GUIDE

KEEPING BABIES AND CHILDREN HEALTHY

A parents' practical handbook to common ailments

Bernard Valman, MD

Foreword by Professor V A Fulginiti, MD,
Editor, American Journal of Diseases of Children, Tucson

Arco Publishing, Inc.
New York

To Thea, my wife and Nadia and Martin our children from whom I
learned how parents feel about their own children

Published in 1985 by Arco Publishing, Inc.
215 Park Avenue South, New York, NY 10003

© H. B. Valman 1985

First published in the United Kingdom in 1985
by Martin Dunitz Ltd, London

Library of Congress Cataloging in Publication Data
Valman, H. B. (Hyman Bernard).
  Keeping babies and children healthy.

  (Positive health guide)
  Includes index.
  1. Children—Care and hygiene.   2. Infants—Care and
hygiene.   3. Pediatrics—Popular works.   I. Title.
II. Series   [DNLM: 1. Child Care—popular works.
2. Infant Care—popular works.   3. Pediatrics—popular
works.   WS 113 V196k]
RJ61.V342 1985   649'.4   84–25759
ISBN 0-668-05809-9
ISBN 0-668-05811-0 (pbk)

Phototypeset in Garamond by Input Typesetting Ltd, London
Printed by Toppan Printing Company (S) Pte Ltd, Singapore

CONTENTS

FOREWORD

Professor V A Fulginiti, MD
Editor, American Journal of Diseases in Children,
Tucson

Of all life's challenges, that of rearing children poses one of the most difficult and, at the same time, enjoyable endeavors. Many parents, faced with this enormous task, find there are many questions that arise in the daily care of their new infant. Further, as the infant grows, additional questions, concerns, worries and curiosities occur for which the parents may have had no prior knowledge or experience. Often parents turn to well-meaning relatives and friends for answers and advice, thinking their queries too trivial to bring to the attention of the physician caring for their child. Folklore, myth, misinterpreted experience and misinformation may be provided to such parents from these sources and from those in the popular media, which parents also turn to for explanation and comfort. This book by Dr Bernard Valman is an effort to supply a fully informed view on many of the common ailments that may afflict growing children in their first seven years of life.

Parents and physicians alike should welcome this text because it correctly anticipates the majority of the questions likely to arise in the parents' minds or in the actual experience of their child. Not only does Dr Valman include the myriad of common concerns, he does so in lucid lay language which is straightforward and non-condescending. One admires the precision with which he uses language in order to instruct, illustrate and otherwise supply information to his readers.

The challenge of child rearing in these critical first few years of life will be made more enjoyable and less difficult for parents who use this book to assist them in the fruitful activity of raising their child with a minimum of unnecessary anxiety and a maximum of solid fact.

INTRODUCTION

From listening and talking to parents who visit my pediatric unit, I have come to realize how important it is to parents to have all the details about the ailments their children may be suffering from – the symptoms, diagnosis, treatment and complications. In this book I have attempted to give a practical account of these common ailments, from the newborn baby to children of 7 years of age, and how parents can contribute to remedying them.

Illness naturally makes parents anxious about their children. This anxiety will be provoked several times in childhood by difficulties with feeding, sleeping and teething; common infectious diseases, skin ailments, fever, eye, ear, throat infections, delayed or slow development – to name but a few. A heightened awareness will guarantee the healthy life of a baby or child who is dependent, at this early age, on his parents. It is a strong, positive attitude; 'fussy' mothers do not exist so no symptoms should be attributed to a mother's anxiety for her child. But this anxiety can be an enormous worry for parents all the same.

From average figures, you can see just how common these ailments are and why every parent should be prepared to deal with them:
Each baby born will have an average of six nose or throat infections and two or three ear infections each pre-school year; in the 5 year-old age group, 7 per cent of children have had at least one convulsion, 5 per cent have a squint; by 7 years old, 16 per cent of children have had their tonsils and adenoids removed, 10 per cent have eczema, asthma or hayfever, 5 per cent will be receiving special schooling, 10 per cent have recurrent abdominal pain; every child will also catch one or more of the common infectious diseases during childhood.

Much of the information on ailments may be passed down from one generation to another, from neighbors and friends and although it can be helpful, it is sometimes quite wrong. With the information in this book, you will be able to act positively, quickly and effectively and feel confident that what you are doing is correct.

I have selected the topics which I know worry parents most, especially mothers with small babies and first-time mothers. I have devoted more space to those problems that affect a large number of babies and children and can be difficult to treat. I have given additional information on medical treatment so that parents have some idea of what to expect the doctor to do and say. Parents will also get some insight into how to make correct diagnoses themselves and how to treat the minor ailments at home.

You may have had the experience of sitting up all night with a crying baby trying to decide whether to feed him again, to telephone your mother or call the doctor. I hope this book will help you to make that decision. It is not intended to be a substitute for your doctor but it will help you to use his help more effectively and appropriately.

Firstly, I want to describe the problems of the newborn baby and how they can be overcome; and then move into the ailments that are common in the first months of life.

At risk of being branded chauvinist, we have referred to babies and children in the text by the masculine pronoun – but this is purely for ease of style and simplicity of reading. It in no way reflects a higher regard for one sex than the other.

Throughout the text, most drugs are referred to by their generic (pharmaceutical) names only. A table of British, American, Canadian and Australian trade names has been included at the end of the book.

1. YOUR NEWBORN BABY

What your newborn baby can do

A normal newborn infant can see, hear, and appreciate pain immediately after birth, even if his mother has been given a strong sedative, such as pethidine, during the delivery. During the hour after birth your baby will often be wide awake, looking for a feed before going to sleep for a few hours.

Seeing

It is a widely believed fallacy that babies cannot see until they are six weeks old, and is often the reason why some mothers do not give their newborns the eye-to-eye contact they need. In fact, the distance between the eyes of the mother and the baby when the mother is breast-feeding is the distance at which newborns can best focus on objects. This eye-to-eye contact supplies the first means of communication between mother and baby, and is important in the creation of the loving bond between them.

If you dangle a brightly coloured object about 12 in (30 cm) in front of your newborn baby, he will become alert, frown and gradually try to focus on the object. He will stare at it intently and will follow the object with short jerky movements of his eyes if you move it slowly from side to side. Your newborn is also sensitive to the intensity of light and will shut his eyes tightly and keep them shut if a bright light is turned on. Research has shown that he can discriminate shapes and patterns and arrangements of lines from birth.

Hearing

Newborn babies respond to sound by blinking, jerking their limbs or drawing in breath, or they may stop feeding. Mothers often speak to their babies in high-pitched tones and babies respond more consistently to their mother's than to their father's voice. Analysis of research films has shown that both the listener and speaker are moving in time to the words of the speaker, creating a type of dance. As the mother pauses for breath, for example, her baby may raise an eyebrow or lower a foot. The mother will notice these responses and this may encourage her to continue speaking. Within a few days of birth your baby may mimic your gestures such as sticking out your tongue or opening your mouth.

Some first-time mothers understandably feel a little foolish when they talk to their babies, and may be at a loss for words, knowing that what they say is not being understood. Of course, it is the tone of your voice that is important to your baby, rather than the actual words you are using. Try giving your baby a running commentary on what you are doing, but remember to pause and give your baby a chance to respond in his own way. Mothers who speak to their babies from birth help to build up the bond of affection that is begun with the first physical and eye-to-eye contact. You will also be encouraging the development of these methods of communication which precede and lead to speech (see pages 37 and 40). If your newborn baby does not look at objects in the way that I have just described, mention this to the doctor who gives your baby his first checkup after leaving the hospital. He or she will recommend further investigations if they think there is any cause for concern.

Feeding problems

In the first few days after birth babies lose a little weight – up to 10 per cent of their birth weight in five days. Full-term infants usually regain their birth weight between the seventh and tenth day, and thereafter should gain around $3/_4$–$1^1/_2$ oz (20–40 g) per day for the next 100 days. You can check your baby's progress at home on a growth chart (see Chapter 2), which is the best guide to making sure that he is receiving the correct amount of milk.

Breast-feeding
On average, around 50–80 per cent of babies in North America are now breast-fed initially, and about half this number are still breast-feeding after three months. There are, though, large regional variations in these figures. At the hospital where I work, for instance, around nine mothers out of ten breast-feed, while in some areas in Britain only four babies out of ten are breast-fed.

The advantages Breast-feeding has the advantage over bottle-feeding in that the fat and protein of breast milk are more completely absorbed into the baby's system than those of bottle milk. The chemical composition of breast milk varies during the feed, and although we still do not understand the significance of these changes they may result in differences in body composition, so that a breast-fed baby's body tissues are slightly different than if he had been fed on bottled milk. As yet no one has proved whether these differences are good or bad for the newborn's health. But if you want everything to be as natural as possible for your baby, there is now scientific backing for the old saying, 'we are what we eat.' In addition, breast milk contains substances which may protect your baby against infections. Gastroenteritis, for example, is extremely rare in breast-fed babies (see Chapter 5). Furthermore, if you give your baby breast milk exclusively for the first six months of life without the occasional night of bottle milk, you may be helping to lessen the risk of his developing a so-called allergic reaction to cow's milk protein (see Chapter 5).

Breast-feeding also plays an important part in mother-infant attachment or bonding. The close contact and intimacy, and often supreme enjoyment, of breast-feeding provide the best feedback between mother and baby.

Many a mother who starts to breast-feed feels insecure and inadequate at first and is only too glad to change to bottle-feeding whenever the slightest difficulty arises. It is at this point that she needs to be given sympathy, understanding and skill, from both the baby's father and the nursing staff, to encourage her to persevere with breast-feeding and gain confidence in handling her own baby. It takes time to pick up these basic skills of motherhood. They are not, as is popularly believed, purely a matter of instinct.

Developing a feeding pattern   A normal newborn baby should be put to the breast for a few minutes on each side, preferably immediately after or a few hours after birth. Only a small amount of yellow, antibody-rich liquid called colostrum is obtained at first, but the infant's sucking soon stimulates the production of more colostrum. Some infants are reluctant to take the nipple initially, but this is a common occurrence and should not put you off breast-feeding. A few days' perseverance may be necessary before your baby loses his reluctance. About three to four days after birth colostrum gives way to mature breast milk.

During the first week and probably later your baby will consume most of the volume and nutrients of his feed within the first four minutes. So during the early days there is little to be gained from breast-feeding for more than ten minutes on each side. Overlong breast-feeds tend to make both mother and baby tired and tense. Try ending his feed with a little previously boiled and cooled water if he still seems thirsty.

The most satisfactory method of breast feeding is 'on demand'. Babies commonly feed every two or three hours during the first few weeks and these frequent feeds are a powerful stimulus to produce more milk. Infants who are fed on demand to start with usually settle down of their own accord to a regular schedule after a few weeks.

After the fourth day, if your baby appears to be hungry after a feed or is progressively losing weight, the doctor might consider trying a period of test feeding. Your baby will be weighed, without changing his diaper or clothes before and after each feed during a twenty-four-hour period. If he is not getting enough milk, putting him to the breast more frequently may stimulate increased production of milk in the early days, or the deficit may be made up with a bottle feed – this is called complementary feeding.

If he is given extra water, a full-term baby with a good birth weight can tolerate a degree of underfeeding without harm for several days, until the mother's milk supply increases to a satisfactory level.

Complementary feeds are rarely necessary in the first five days, after this they should only be used when absolutely necessary. The feel of the bottle nipple is quite different from that of the mother's nipple, and when your baby is accustomed to drinking milk from one it may be difficult to persuade him to take from the other. Also, your baby will use a different sucking technique with a bottle. He can let air into the bottle at intervals to help the milk flow more freely than if he was breast-feeding. Finding it easier to feed from a bottle, he may then not be so keen to return to the breast. By giving complementary bottle feeds you will reduce your baby's appetite for breast milk. If he does not empty your breast at each feed, your supply of milk will begin to run down.

Breast-fed babies should receive vitamin supplements, particularly vitamin D, until the age of two years. These are available without prescription, and your pharmacist will be able to advise you on which preparations are most suitable.

Can you take drugs?   A breast-feeding mother should only take essential drugs prescribed by her physician. Most of these are excreted in the milk in insignificant amounts, so your doctor will not advise you to stop breast-feeding unless there is a special reason. Occasional doses of the following drugs pass into the milk in minute amounts and should not affect your baby:

- Aspirin: for pain
- Acetaminophen: for pain
- Senna: for constipation
- Steroids: for asthma
- Barbiturates: for insomnia
- Phenytoin: for epilepsy
- Digoxin: for heart trouble
- Warfarin: for blood clotting in the veins.

The estrogen hormones contained in the oral contraceptive pill may reduce a breast-feeding mother's milk supply, but the progesterone-only pill is an effective contraceptive and has no effect on lactation. Interestingly, breast-feeding itself has a contraceptive effect, but it is not 100 per cent effective, and is only significant if your baby suckles frequently and feeds exclusively on breast milk. The effect is strongest in the first three months after birth. If you are taking any other type of drug, seek further advice from your doctor.

When it would be better not to breast-feed   Severe postnatal depression is not necessarily a reason in itself to stop breast-feeding. Indeed, a depressed mother may feel even more despondent if she is advised not to continue. But if her doctor thinks that a course of antidepressant drug therapy may be necessary, this would be one of the few reasons why breast-feeding would be inadvisable. Therefore the mother and her doctor must discuss the situation carefully and decide whether to continue with breast-feeding without antidepressant drugs, or vice-versa.

Some women have a revulsion to the idea of breast-feeding, and it would be a mistake for anyone to try to persuade them to start.

A few mothers develop a severely cracked nipple while breast-feeding and should stop feeding from the affected side until the nipple heals (see below). Occasionally, an abscess forms in a nursing mother's breast, which can be recognized by a tender, red area on the skin. Your doctor will prescribe a course of antibiotics for this, and feeding can be continued from the affected breast.

Problems with breast-feeding Occasionally the supply of breast milk builds up too slowly on the first and second days after birth. This can be stimulated and increased by putting your baby to the breast more frequently, perhaps every two hours.

On the fourth or fifth day, when you have a plentiful supply of breast milk, your baby may take up to eight feeds or more a day. Loose green stools after each feed are common at this stage and perfectly normal. Conversely, some thriving breast-fed infants pass stools only once a week when they reach the age of a few weeks. These stools are usually of normal consistency and the baby does not cry with pain when passing them. This is not due to constipation and requires no treatment. In fact, breast-fed babies are rarely constipated. Constipation is an altered bowel habit when the infant is passing harder and less frequent stools than previously, and in the first months of life usually only affects bottle-fed babies (see later in this chapter).

Cracked nipple (see above) is usually due to placing your baby incorrectly on the nipple so that the whole of the brown area (areola) is *not* in his mouth. To prevent this, make sure he sucks on the whole areola. This spreads the pressure of his sucking over a wider area and puts less strain on the nipple itself. Pulling the infant off your breast abruptly is another cause of cracked nipple. This can be avoided by placing your little finger in your baby's mouth and opening it slightly before removing the nipple. If your nipple is cracked you should take your baby off that breast for a day or two and apply a soothing ointment, such as lanolin, on the affected nipple every few hours. There is no advantage for healing or prevention in using an antiseptic nipple spray.

Feeding on demand usually prevents breast engorgement – an aching swelling of the breast due to its containing too much milk. This can occur towards the end of the first week of your baby's life and may prevent the

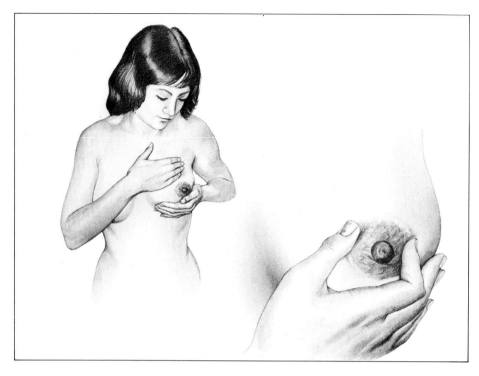

You can find relief from breast engorgement by taking a warm bath and expressing the milk by hand.

milk from flowing from the nipple. The discomfort can easily be alleviated by expressing the surplus milk after feeding, preferably with an electric breast pump (now available in most hospitals). If your breasts do become engorged you will need the doctor's or midwife's help. Taking two acetaminophen pills at recommended intervals will ease the discomfort, which should not last more than a couple of days. If you are at home, taking a warm bath and expressing the milk by hand may help to reduce the swelling (see diagram above).

During the first feed of the morning, milk may spurt quickly from your breast and if your baby is ravenous he may swallow excessive air. If he is not properly burped the air may be brought up later with a little of the milk. This regurgitation is often accompanied by severe crying. This problem can be avoided by expressing the first ounce or so of milk by hand. The excess milk can be given to your infant later if he is still hungry after he has emptied your breasts. The best method to bring up air after a feed is to place your baby on his stomach, with his head higher than his feet and turned to one side. You can do this simply by placing some blankets under the head end of his crib or carrier.

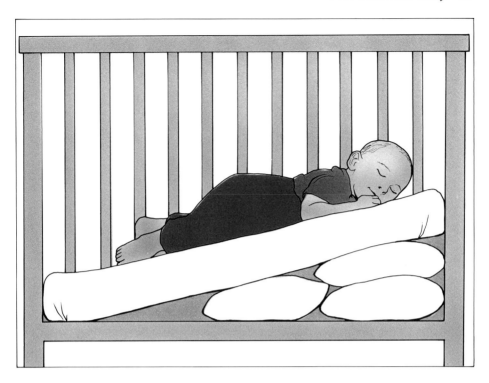

Burping position. Raise your baby's head higher than his feet by placing blankets or cushions under the crib mattress.

Bottle-feeding

All the powdered and liquid cows' milk preparations have a chemical composition similar to that of breast milk and contain your baby's complete vitamin requirements. Bottle-feeding, though, gives your baby no immunity to infection and there is an increased risk of his picking up an infection such as gastroenteritis (see Chapter 5) through inadequately sterilized bottles and feeding equipment.

Bottles must always be sterilized before use. The simplest method is to immerse them completely in a commercially available sterilizing solution. Always check there are no air bubbles trapped in bottles or nipples, as any area not in contact with the solution will not be sterilized. Before being immersed, the nipple should be rubbed inside and out with table salt and rinsed out with water.

The instructions on each packet for making up bottle-milk must be followed and the powder should be measured accurately, avoiding heaped or packed scoops, which will tend to make your baby put on too much weight.

If you make up feeds for a twenty-four-hour period you should store them in the refrigerator, as milk left for a long period at room temperature makes an ideal breeding ground for germs such as the bacteria which cause gastroenteritis.

Bottle-milk should be given at room temperature. If stored in the refrigerator, you can stand the bottle on the table for ten minutes or so to warm up the milk. Before putting the nipple into your baby's mouth the temperature of the milk should be checked by allowing a few drops to fall on the back of your hand.

Feeds can be given on demand, or three or four hourly. With the modern milk preparations most babies need to be fed every three hours but, as I have said, the milk must not be made up to a stronger concentration than that recommended on the packet.

A normal full-term baby should receive $1/2$ fl oz milk per lb body weight (30 ml per kg) during the first day of feeding by bottle. Feeds should be increased by $1/3$ fl oz per lb (20 ml per kg) each day until a maximum of $2^{1}/_{2}$ fl oz per lb (150 ml per kg) is reached on the seventh day of feeding. If for any reason your baby needs more fluid, water can be added to the feeds to increase the volume to the maximum requirement for day seven.

Problems with bottle feeding   If the hole in the nipple is too small your baby may swallow excessive air during the feed and bring it up later with milk accompanied by bouts of crying. Watch the rate at which the drops of milk are formed when the bottle is tipped up. They should follow each other quickly but should not form a continuous stream. If the hole is too small, it can be enlarged with a hot sewing needle which has been held in a flame. When buying nipples make sure they have the medium-size holes. Another way in which your baby might swallow too much air while feeding is if you allow air as well as milk to pass through the nipple. Holding the bottle at an angle steep enough for the milk to fill the nipple completely will prevent this problem.

If your baby is not putting on weight as fast as he should (see next chapter) he needs more frequent or larger feeds. If the weather is hot and he is not receiving extra water he may be thirsty and you should offer him the equivalent of two feeds of previously boiled water per day in addition to his normal milk feeds. Giving extra water will also help if your baby is straining to pass hard, infrequent stools. Constipation in bottle-fed newborns should not be treated with laxatives.

Infants are rarely too greedy, but if yours is, you should seek advice from your doctor on the possibility of him or her prescribing a mild sedative.

If your baby has fed normally before, and suddenly stops feeding, this may be a symptom of underlying illness, and he should be seen by your doctor. When a newborn has a cold his nose may become temporarily blocked with mucus, making it difficult for him to feed. Your doctor may give salt solution nose drops to help clear the nasal congestion.

A few bottle-fed babies are affected by an infection called thrush, or candidiasis. Thrush produces white patches on the tongue and inside the mouth which become sore and make it painful to feed. Your doctor will prescribe antibiotic drops, such as nystatin, which can be squirted into the mouth with a needleless syringe, or plastic dropper or pipette. The full course of antibiotics must be given and the infection usually clears up after about a week. Thrush is mainly transmitted to a baby at birth from the mother via the birth canal or via hands, nipples or breasts at feeding time; this is why it is so important to thoroughly wash your hands before feeding your baby.

Vomiting in the newborn

Vomiting is the forceful expulsion of the stomach's contents through the mouth. Parents often confuse vomiting with spitting up, or regurgitation, which is the effortless bringing up of small amounts of milk during and between feeds, usually accompanied by air. If the milk dribbles down your baby's chest it is likely to be spitting up rather than vomiting. As I mentioned previously, babies often bring up small amounts of milk with air after a feed and this is no cause for concern. It is a popular fallacy that vomiting or spitting up are due to the baby's milk – either breast or bottled – not being suitable.

If an infant who has not previously vomited begins to vomit he should be seen by a doctor as this may be a sign of an infection such as a urinary tract infection, which will need treatment with antibiotics (see Chapter 5). Gastroenteritis sometimes begins in this way, with diarrhea following after a day or two. This infection can be dangerous in newborns because without proper treatment they can suffer serious loss of body fluids. I discuss the treatment of gastroenteritis in detail in Chapter 5.

Some infants regurgitate persistently until they start to stand and walk, and this is believed to be due to weakness of the circular muscle at the lower end of the gullet where it joins the stomach. To help overcome this problem you can try the following methods. Feed your baby in the upright position strapped into a canvas chair suitable for newborns (see photograph overleaf); he should remain there for half an hour after a feed. Another way is to ensure that all the air is brought up shortly after a feed by placing your baby on his stomach as described on page 14. The third possibility is to thicken his feed with powdered carob seed flour (Carobel). Recurrent regurgitation is very common and although it is exhausting to carry out so much washing, the problem will resolve spontaneously by the time your child reaches the age of a year. As I have already mentioned, if you bottle-feed your baby it is important to remember that if the hole in the nipple is too small or the bottle is not tipped high enough he will swallow air and regurgitate it with milk.

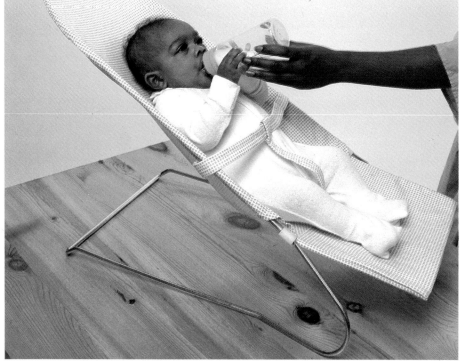

To help prevent vomiting, bottle-feed your baby in an upright position, strapped into a canvas chair.

If your baby's vomit is yellowish (bile-stained), or contains blood you should contact a doctor immediately, as this may be a sign that he has a serious intestinal problem such as intussusception (see Chapter 5).

Pyloric stenosis

This condition, which affects only 0.3 per cent of babies, is a thickening of the wall of the stomach where it joins the beginning of the small intestine. This thickening narrows the tube down which food passes to the intestine. Food accumulates in the stomach and then forceful vomiting occurs, vomit being projected several feet from the infant. The vomiting usually begins in the second or third week of life and your baby may lose weight due to loss of body fluids and fat. If he passes much less urine than usual this is due to the dehydration.

Your baby should be seen by a doctor without delay, and he will attempt to feel the thickening of the stomach by examining your infant during a feed. If the diagnosis is confirmed a small operation is needed to reduce the obstruction produced by the thick muscle. Your baby will probably only need to be in the hospital for forty-eight hours. He needs no special diet after the operation and the wound should heal up after about ten days. There should be no dressings to be changed. This treatment completely cures pyloric stenosis.

Jaundice

Jaundice is a yellow colouring of the skin and whites of the eyes by a high concentration of a pigment in the blood called bilirubin. Around one-third of newborn babies are affected by jaundice, its cause in nearly all cases being a build-up of pigment due to inability of the immature liver to cope with the large number of red blood cells that are normally destroyed shortly after birth. This common type of jaundice usually starts more than twenty-four hours after birth and reaches its highest level on the fourth or fifth day.

What can be done?
Most babies with jaundice need no treatment, but many become a little sluggish and reluctant to feed. It is important to encourage them to take as much fluid as possible, by offering water after a milk feed, as the more they drink the more bilirubin pigment is excreted from their system.

Babies who have moderate jaundice may be given a painless blood test to find out the level of bilirubin. A small number of these infants may then be given phototherapy for two or three days in the special care unit (see the end of this chapter) or in your ward. This is simply a method of bathing your baby in fluorescent light to change the bilirubin into a harmless, colourless chemical. During phototherapy your baby's eyes will be shielded with eye pads held in place with tube gauze.

Rarely the level of bilirubin in the blood is found to be high enough to be a serious risk to your baby's health. He will then need a complete exchange blood transfusion to prevent further problems. The transfusion is a painless procedure which takes around two to three hours. This type of jaundice is usually caused by an incompatibility between a baby's rhesus positive blood and his mother's rhesus negative blood. Although one baby in ten has the potential for this type of incompatibility, preventive medical techniques have made the problem much less common than it used to be.

If your baby seems to be ill as well as jaundiced, this may be due to an infection such as a urinary tract or blood infection. The doctor will take blood and urine samples for testing, and if the results confirm the presence of an infection, your baby will be prescribed a course of antibiotics to clear up the problem.

Occasionally in breast-fed babies jaundice persists at a very low level for two or three months. If jaundice with no other accompanying symptoms continues for longer than ten days in a full-term baby, blood and urine tests will be performed to rule out other rare causes such as an underactive thyroid gland. If all these tests are negative you can continue breast-feeding, as these very low levels of bilirubin will have no effect on your baby. In this situation there is no need to worry throughout the first few months that the bilirubin in your baby's blood might suddenly rise to dangerous levels, since once a low level has been reached, it will not bounce up again (except perhaps briefly after phototherapy, after which the level settles to normal). The jaundice will clear up in time of its own accord. Interestingly, a high level of the hormone progesterone has been found in the milk of some mothers whose babies have mild jaundice for several weeks after birth.

Very rarely jaundice that starts more than twenty-four hours after birth can be a sign of a serious underlying condition, either an infection of the liver – hepatitis (see page 64) – or absence of the bile ducts which carry bile away from the liver to the gall bladder and intestine. If there is a bile duct problem, your baby will pass stools as white as paper, and an operation may be necessary to try to rectify the problem. To put this type of jaundice into reassuring perspective, I would expect to see only one such case in twenty years' work as a pediatrician.

Eye problems in the newborn

Pink eye (conjunctivitis)

Chemicals such as chlorhexidene used in swabbing the mother during delivery may affect the thin transparent membrane, or conjunctiva, covering a baby's eye at birth. This may cause mild inflammation and a sticky eye which gets better by itself without treatment within a day or two. You can clean the closed eyelids with cotton wool which has been moistened with cooled boiled water. If there is yellow discharge from the eye it is likely that a bacterial infection is present and the doctor will prescribe an antibiotic ointment to be applied to both eyes three times daily for a week. The ointment comes in a tube with a fine nozzle at one end. The technique of applying the ointment is as follows: while your baby is asleep, squeeze out a thin strip along his upper eyelid, just above the eyelashes. Start from the inside edge of the eye and move outwards, taking care not to touch the surface of his eye or eyelid with the nozzle. Do ask the nurse for help at first if you do not feel confident enough to do this.

Before prescribing a particular antibiotic the doctor may take a swab to find out exactly which type of bacteria is responsible. If the condition has not cleared up within a week, make sure your baby is seen again by a doctor.

Watering eye
If your baby's eye waters persistently with clear fluid, his tear duct is probably blocked. This causes no discomfort, so no action is required at least until the age of a year, when your infant can be seen by an eye surgeon. Most eye surgeons prefer to take no action even at this stage because the condition stops by itself in virtually all infants before they reach eighteen months.

If at any time you notice repeated yellow discharge from the eye, take your baby to the doctor. He or she will take an eye swab for examination in a laboratory to determine the most suitable antibiotic ointment.

Is your baby normal?

Along with the joy of your baby's birth, there is a natural anxiety about whether he is perfectly normal and healthy. In this section I look first at some of the normal physical variations that can occur in newborn babies, and then at some of the more common minor abnormalities and how you can cope with them.

Normal variations

The caput   Many babies have a soft swelling, called the caput, over the part of the head which was born first. This is an accumulation of fluids under the skin caused by the normal pressure exerted on the head during labour. It disappears of its own accord in a few days.

Bruising   A few babies have a swelling on one side of the top of the head, which has the medical name cephalhaematoma. This is a small harmless bruise under the skin and, like the caput, occurs following normal delivery. Sometimes three to four weeks after birth a hard rim can be felt round the edge of the bruise. The swelling usually disappears without treatment in two or three months but sometimes a hard bony swelling may persist for several months.

'Stork marks'   Most babies have some fine red lines on the upper eyelid, and on the back of the head at the hairline. These lines, called 'stork marks', disappear by the age of a year.

Hair   It is common for a newborn's fine hair to fall out after a few weeks or months and it will soon be replaced by new hair of the adult type.

Spots   Most newborn infants have whitish-yellow pinhead size spots on the nose and the surrounding part of the cheeks. These disappear without treatment but may reappear during the first few months of life.

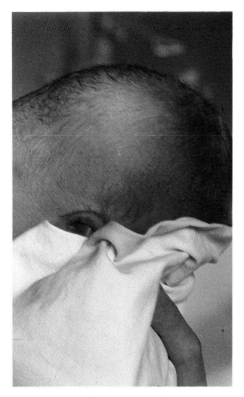

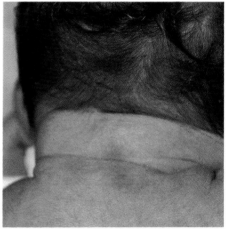

The caput. It will disappear of its own accord a few days after birth.

'Stork marks' – a normal variation at birth which usually disappears by the age of one.

Enlarged breasts   About 50 per cent of newborn babies, whether girls or boys, have some swelling of the breasts. This may last for several weeks. No treatment is required and you shouldn't try to squeeze the breasts. At the beginning of pregnancy the mother's breasts enlarge in response to the release of certain hormones from the ovaries. During pregnancy some of these hormones pass into the baby's bloodstream through the umbilical cord and later cause a similar enlargement of the baby's breasts.

Vaginal discharge   A few days after birth some girls have a small amount of mucous discharge from the vagina and occasionally slight bleeding with it. This is again due to the mother's hormones circulating in the baby's blood and no treatment is needed.

Coping with minor abnormalities
Around 3–4 per cent of babies are born with some degree of abnormality. Fortunately, many of these abnormalities can now be treated so effectively

that they cause few, if any, problems for the child as he grows up.

We do not know the cause of most abnormalities. But routine prenatal investigations, such as blood tests and ultrasound scans, may detect a severe abnormality soon enough after conception to allow parents and doctor to discuss the possibility of terminating the pregnancy. The following are some of the possible causes of abnormalities in babies:

- **Heredity** If you know of any abnormalities in other members of your family, it is wise to discuss these with your doctor either before conception or as early in pregnancy as possible.
- **Drugs** Certain types of drugs taken in pregnancy, especially during the first three months, can adversely affect the fetus. These include alcohol in excess and nicotine from tobacco. It is very important to discuss with your doctor the taking of any drugs during pregnancy. You should also give up smoking, and cut out, or at least cut down on alcohol.
- **Infection** Despite being a mild disease for the mother, German measles (rubella) can cause serious abnormalities in the fetus if contracted during the first twelve weeks of pregnancy. All young girls should be immunized to avoid this happening to them in later life (see Chapter 3).
- **Mother's age** The risk of having a baby with an abnormality does increase with the mother's age, especially for Down's syndrome or so-called Mongolism. For this reason pregnant women over forty may be advised to have the amniocentesis test, which is used to identify conditions such as Down's syndrome in the fetus. The test involves obtaining and analysing some of the fetus's skin cells which have been shed into the surrounding amniotic fluid in the womb.

The following are some of the commonest minor abnormalities affecting babies at or shortly after birth:

The strawberry mark starts as a tiny red spot and grows rapidly for several weeks until it has a raised, red appearance with tiny white spots which look like the seeds of a strawberry. These marks are common in premature babies. They may occur anywhere on the body but cause no symptoms, except on the eyelids, where they may prevent easy opening of the eyes and need treatment. Strawberry marks grow, often rapidly, for three to nine months, but at least 90 per cent resolve by themselves, either completely or partially. Improvement usually begins at six to nine months and is complete in half the children affected by the age of five, and in 70 per cent by the age of seven years. In 80 per cent of cases these marks disappear completely.

The port-wine stain is far less common than the strawberry mark. It is not raised and may be extensive. It does not disappear, but the skin texture remains normal. If it is present on the face a cosmetic masking cream recommended by your doctor or pharmacist can be used to hide the stain.

Neonatal urticaria consists of blotchy, ill-defined areas of redness surrounding white or yellow raised spots which may resemble septic spots. It is very common and usually appears on the second day of life. In most affected infants it clears within forty-eight hours. The spots tend to disappear within a few hours, to be replaced by others elsewhere.

Mongolian blue spots are patchy build-ups of pigment, especially over the buttocks and lower back in babies of races with pigmented skins. They are common in infants of African or Mongolian descent, but also occur in Italian and Greek babies. They look very like bruises and become less obvious as the skin darkens.

Dislocated and dislocatable hip   In the first two days of life about 1 in 200 babies has this type of hip abnormality. The problem is more common in girls and after the breech position at birth. A previous member of the family may have had the same condition. It is usually not possible for the mother to detect an abnormality of the hip at this stage, but all newborn infants are examined at some time during the first three days by the midwife or doctor in order to detect this condition.

Early treatment is simple and usually effective. It consists of holding the hips in a good position with the thighs flexed by means of a padded light-metal splint for two to three months. This helps the head of the thigh bone to mold a normal socket for itself in the hip. The splinting will be supervised by an orthopedic surgeon every one or two weeks.

Once the splint is in place you should try to continue with breast-feeding if you began feeding your baby this way. The position of his legs may make this awkward at first but most mothers soon get used to it. You should wash your baby without removing the splint. You can insert wads of cotton wool between the splint and your baby's skin at places where chaffing is likely to occur. These should be replaced without disturbing the splint if they become dirty or wet. When dressing your baby, put his clothes on over the splint, not under it. When the splint is eventually removed your efforts will almost certainly be rewarded as the hips are usually normal.

Club-foot   This condition affects around 7 babies in 10,000. It is a mis-shaping of the foot, which is generally due to one of two causes. The commonest and least problematic is a muscular imbalance due to the cramped position of the fetus's feet in the womb before birth. If the condition is due solely to muscular imbalance it should be possible to bend the foot so that its upper surface touches the shin. The shape of the foot usually returns to normal within a few weeks but it may be possible to speed up this process by gently manipulating the foot through its whole range of movements after each feed.

In contrast, if there is a bony abnormality of the foot, the foot's range of movements will be restricted and an orthopedic specialist will treat the foot with manipulation and strapping within twenty-four hours of birth. In many cases early strapping alone is successful but a series of plastercasts may be needed later or, less commonly, an operation.

Extra fingers and toes are rare but are often hereditary and vary from an apparently normal finger to a skin tag. The latter can be tied off painlessly with a sterile silk thread by the doctor or midwife and will separate after about a week. An extra finger or toe which looks like a normal digit should be removed by a plastic surgeon, usually when your child is a few years of age.

Cleft lip and palate   Failure of the two halves of either the upper lip or palate to join before birth occurs in around 1 in every 1,000 babies. Parents are often severely disturbed by the appearance of their baby's cleft lip, but may be reassured by seeing photographs of similar babies before and after their repair operation. Cleft lip and cleft palate are often associated.

Most infants with a cleft lip or palate feed normally from the breast or bottle despite their abnormality. If there are feeding difficulties, a special nipple, a large normal nipple, a special spade-like spoon, or an ordinary spoon may help.

Cleft lip is usually repaired by plastic surgery at three months and the palate at one year. The value of fitting a plate in the roof of the mouth to cover over the space in the cleft palate before the operation is controversial and should be discussed with the doctor who is treating your baby. Despite excellent operative results children with a cleft palate may be prone to recurrent ear infections (see Chapter 4) and problems with speech development (see Chapter 2). Parents should be on the alert for these and should seek qualified advice if they occur.

Umbilical hernia   A large swelling in the region of the navel is most common in African infants or West Indians of African descent. No treatment is needed, as the hernia usually disappears of its own accord by the age of three years, although for West Indian infants it may take another three years.

Heart problems   The most common heart problem in babies is a murmur, or odd heart sound, discovered with a stethoscope during a routine examination, either in the newborn period or later on in life during an acute illness. The majority of murmurs will not be due to a structural abnormality of the heart but will be found to be a variation on the normal sounds of blood flowing through the tubes of the heart. In some children more noise

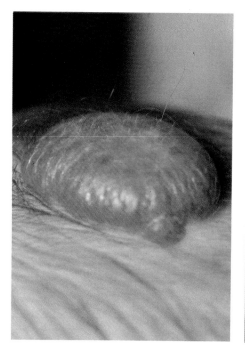

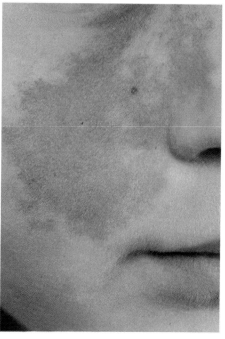

A strawberry mark is a common minor abnormality, particularly in premature babies.

There are some excellent cosmetic masking creams on the market for hiding a port-wine stain.

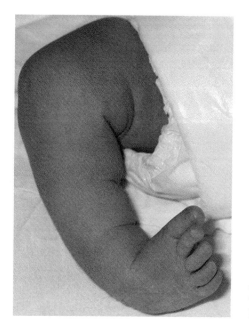

A structural club-foot where the top of the foot cannot be made to touch the baby's shin.

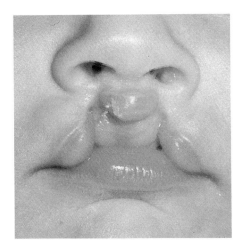

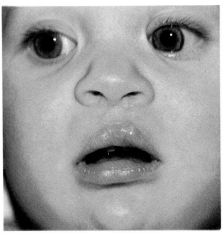

A cleft lip before plastic surgery.

A cleft lip after surgery. The baby's appearance is now completely normal.

is produced than in others, similar to the noise in some central heating systems. Once the doctor has excluded any form of heart disease your baby can be considered completely normal and should be treated as such. If a murmur has been noted on one occasion it is likely to be heard again at routine examinations and whenever your child has fever, when it may be more noticeable.

In newborn babies a murmur may be due to late closure of a blood vessel near the heart, which is open before birth and usually closes within the first few days of life. These babies feed and behave normally and when the doctor listens to the chest again after a period of one to three weeks the murmur has usually gone.

Doctors listen to the newborn baby's heart to check, among other things, whether a structural abnormality might be present. Around 1 in every 100 babies has a structural abnormality of the heart – usually the so-called hole in the heart, which is due to failure of one of the partitions of the heart to close before birth. Most of these defects close without treatment before

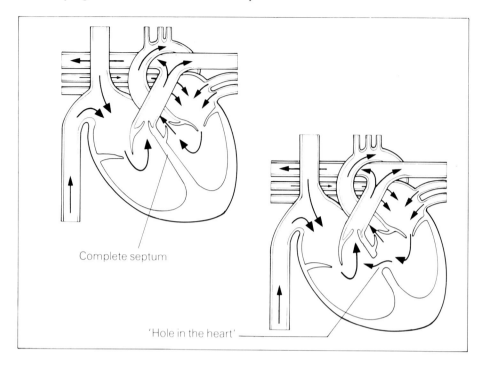

Complete septum

'Hole in the heart'

Most 'hole in the heart' defects close up without treatment.

your child reaches the age of five years. Your child should engage in all the usual activities, and will grow normally whether or not the hole in the heart closes. To make absolutely sure that no structural abnormality is present the doctor may decide to carry out further investigations. These may include an X-ray of the chest, an electrocardiogram (EKG) and an ultrasound scan. The EKG involves taking recordings of the heartbeat from electrodes placed on your baby's limbs and chest. Your baby will not feel any discomfort during this procedure. The ultrasound scan is similar to that given to most mothers during the pregnancy. It is not painful and does not involve X-rays.

If a hole in the heart does not close up eventually, an operation may be needed to stitch a patch of synthetic material over the hole. This is now a very safe operation and your child should have recovered fully about six weeks after it is carried out.

Others   There are of course several other types of congenital abnormalities. I have not described the more serious ones such as Down's syndrome or spina bifida, as if these conditions are to be covered at all, they need to be dealt with in too great a depth for the scope of this book.

A few abnormalities such as undescended testicle and hypospadias – an abnormal position for the opening of the urethra in the penis – I describe under the appropriate headings in Chapter 5.

Special care baby units

Eight to fifteen per cent of newborn babies spend some time in a special care baby unit. Nowadays, many hospitals are equipped with special care facilities, but many are not, and so if necessary mother and baby may be taken to the nearest hospital with a special care baby unit.

These units are designed and equipped for newborn babies who need extra medical and nursing care. This may be necessary for premature babies, babies with breathing difficulties or jaundice (see previously), for newborns recovering from a difficult delivery, or for infants who need special medical tests to find out whether they are ill or not.

The equipment

Incubator   The perspex-covered environment of the incubator allows doctors and nurses to keep a close watch on your baby's unclothed body, while at the same time keeping him warm.

Monitoring   Sophisticated electronic sensors painlessly attached to your baby's skin enable his condition to be measured and displayed without his being touched or disturbed. His heart rate, temperature and breathing rate can all be monitored in this way.

Premature babies occasionally stop breathing for a while, and this pause is called apnoea. An apnoea alarm is part of the incubator's monitoring equipment. If it sounds, a nurse or doctor will quickly stimulate the baby to restart breathing, and no harm will have been done.

Respirator   There are several causes of breathing difficulties in newborns, among them being lung infections, and immaturity of the lungs which leads to very rapid breathing, known as respiratory distress syndrome.

Treatment of breathing difficulties is now very effective, and often involves the use of a respirator which can either assist or completely take over the baby's breathing. The machine supplies oxygen through a tube inserted painlessly into the baby's nose or mouth.

Feeding and contact

Babies in a special care unit will be fed either by a tube through the nose into the stomach or by a drip into a vein. Neither procedure causes discomfort for the baby, but mothers may be disappointed that they cannot

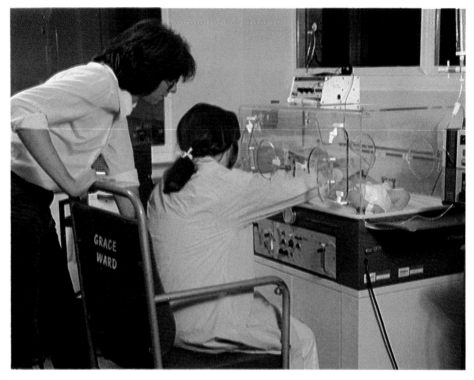

Parents can still touch, stroke and talk to their baby through windows in the side of the incubator.

begin breast-feeding in the normal way. It is possible, though, to express and collect your breast milk, and then have it fed to your baby via the stomach tube. Ask the nursing staff for advice if you wish to do this.

Apart from the worry of your baby having to be in special care, you will also feel that you and your baby are being deprived of the close contact that most mothers, fathers and babies take for granted and enjoy in the first days after birth. But just because your baby is in an incubator does not mean that you must be completely separated. There are windows on the sides of the incubator which you may be allowed to open and through which you can touch, stroke and talk to your baby. As I mentioned at the beginning of this chapter, eye-to-eye contact is very important at this stage. Placing your face close to the incubator's door in front of your baby's face will put you in the best position for your baby to focus on your features. The nursing staff in a special care unit know how important early contact is between parents and baby and will allow you every possible opportunity of being close to your baby at this time.

Babies born very early are usually allowed to leave the special care unit and go home about two weeks before their original expected date of delivery. The majority of premature babies survive and grow up to be normal children even if they are born as much as three months too early.

The newborn, or neonatal, stage is complete a month after your baby's delivery date. In the next chapter I shall be looking at some of the common problems that arise during the first few months after the neonatal period.

2. THE FIRST MONTHS

In this chapter I shall be looking at the aspects of babies' health that most commonly cause concern to parents during the first months of life. These include growth and development, persistent crying, colic, sleeping problems, weaning and teething. Some ailments, such as diarrhea or eczema, may also affect babies during this time, but they are common in older children too, so are covered in later chapters.

Infant growth

The size of the normal baby at birth is determined mainly by his mother's size. The greatest changes in size caused by other hereditary factors, such as his father's stature, take place during the first six months of life. For example, a baby of average size and weight at birth may become above average height and weight within a couple of months if he has a large father and average-size mother. Although children tend eventually to reach a stature between those of their parents, some children take after one parent, grandparent or an even more remote member of the family. All these children are perfectly healthy.

It may be difficult to distinguish these normal adjustments in growth from a growth problem caused either by too much or too little feeding, or illness, especially during the first few months of life. Checking your baby's progress on a growth chart is the best way to confirm whether his growth pattern is normal or not. Using the chart overleaf, you can record details weekly for the first ten weeks, then every two weeks or so. Domestic scales are not accurate enough for weighing young babies, so you will need to have him weighed by your doctor, or buy or rent scales specially designed for weighing babies. Height is difficult to measure accurately in very young babies, but you can measure the head circumference to compare with the weight. You measure the head circumference round the forehead and the back of the head, moving the tape measure up and down until you get the largest measurement. Paper tape measures are accurate but linen tape measures are unsuitable as they stretch and produce inaccurate results.

How to use a growth chart
You will see on the chart overleaf that there are three heavy lines in both the weight and head circumference sections. The center line is the mean,

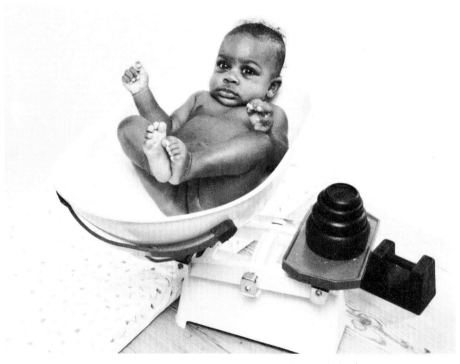

Above: You may be able to rent a set of scales to weigh your baby in.

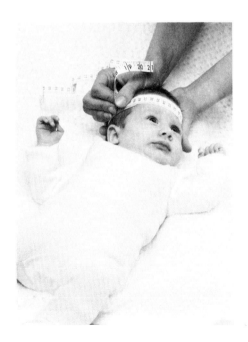

Paper tape measures are more accurate than linen ones for measuring your baby's head circumference because they do not stretch.

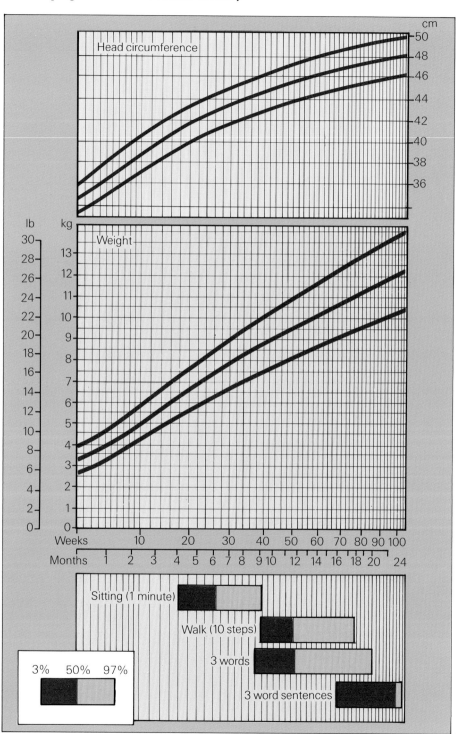

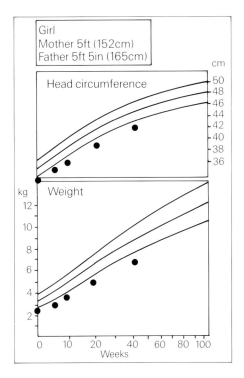

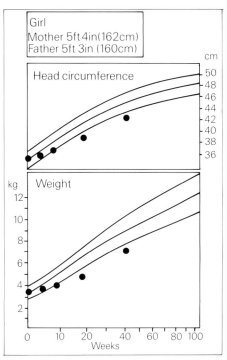

The normal growth chart for a baby with short parents.

The normal growth chart for a baby w̶ẗ̶ʰ̶ a small father.

or average measurement for the baby population as a whole, while the area between the top and bottom lines of each section represents the normal range of weight or head circumference. Only a small proportion of babies will have measurements outside these areas. Weight and head circumference are shown together on the same chart because it is nearly always the relationship between these two measurements that is important when checking for growth problems, rather than the fact that both may be low or high. When both sets of measurements run parallel to each other, your baby's growth is normal.

Let's take a look at some common examples to clarify these points. One of the anxieties about growth I come across most frequently is expressed by short parents who are worried that their baby is not growing or eating

Opposite: Use this chart to record the changes in your baby's weight and head circumference each week. You can also record your baby's development progress over the next 24 months. (3%, 50% and 97% refer to the percentage of the total number of babies).

enough. A glance at the chart on page 35 (*left*) for a baby with short parents shows that although the baby's head circumference and weight are unusually low, they are increasing in parallel – a strong indication that all is well.

Another common cause of worry for parents is when a baby of a medium-size mother and a small (or large) father seems to be gaining too little or too much weight respectively during the first months. Again, the chart on page 35 (*right*) shows that a small father's baby does indeed seem to be gaining weight more slowly than normal, but the head circumference shows an identical slow pattern of development. This indicates that the whole of the baby's size is moving towards that of one of his parents – in this case his father.

The chart below shows an example of a baby failing to thrive due to his mother's insufficient supply of breast milk. As soon as the weight measurement line dropped significantly out of parallel with the head circumference line, I advised the mother to change to bottle-feeding, which quickly brought her baby's weight gain back to a normal pattern. If weight

The growth chart of a baby who failed to thrive as the supply of breast milk was insufficient. When bottle milk was introduced, the growth pattern returned to normal.

The growth chart of an overweight baby.

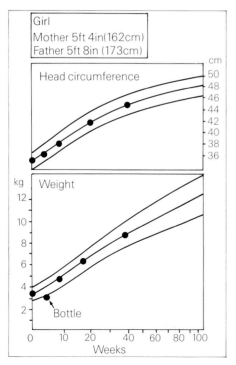

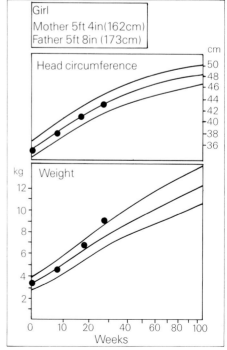

gain drops in this way after solids are introduced, this may be due to an ailment such as celiac disease where food is not absorbed properly from the intestine (see Chapter 5).

A minor illness such as a cold might cause your baby's weight line to dip temporarily. But his normal growth and weight pattern is usually regained within two weeks.

Growth charts can also give you an early warning that your baby is becoming overweight. In the final chart example the baby's weight gain began an upward trend at four months, with no corresponding change on the head circumference line. I discovered that the mother had been over-feeding her baby with newly introduced solid food and had not started to reduce the amount of bottle-fed milk which her baby had been taking before starting on solids. A few weeks after balancing her baby's diet more carefully, his weight gain dropped back into step with the rate of increase of his head circumference.

If you are worried for any reason about your baby's rate of growth then discuss it with your family doctor. In the rare event that he or she considers that there is an underlying medical problem such as celiac disease or a hormonal deficiency, your baby will need to have specialized medical tests and treatment.

Infant development

Among normal infants there is a large difference in the age when they start a particular activity. For example, some normal children start to walk by themselves at the age of nineteen months whereas others start at ten months. Similarly, some infants are speaking only a few words at two years whereas others are talking continuously in sentences by that age. Just because your baby is starting to walk later than your neighbor's does not mean that there is anything wrong with him. Each child is unique and differs from others in his physical, emotional and mental development. Most children are more advanced than average in some fields of development and slower than average in others. Because your child is faster at a certain ability does not mean that his final intelligence will be above average.

Advances in one aspect of development – in talking, for example – tend to happen in spurts. No changes seem to occur for perhaps several months and then suddenly your child may appear to pick up a whole new vocabu-lary within a few days. When your baby is acquiring a new ability such as talking he may well stop progressing in another field such as walking. Girls tend to walk, talk and become dry earlier than boys. Some children

Overleaf: The progressive stages you can expect to see in the development of your baby from 0–20 months.

0–1 MONTH

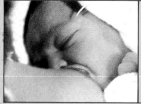 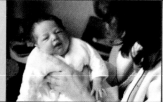 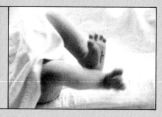

Feed   Look around   Kick

2–4 MONTHS

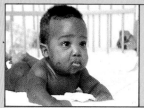 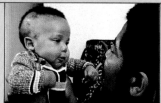 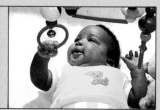

Support himself   Listen and talk   Look at and reach
on his elbows   in his way   towards
                                                 toy over cot

8–12 MONTHS

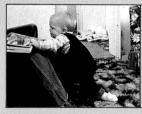 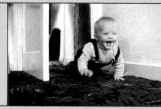 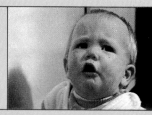

Pull herself up to   Move by crawling, bottom   Make 'mum-mum'
standing   shuffling or rolling   sounds

1-2 MONTHS

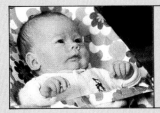 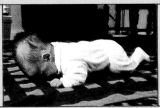 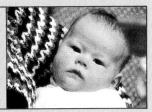

Take interest when supported in chair

Lift head from floor

Focus eyes on people and things

5-10 MONTHS

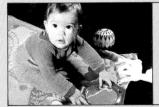 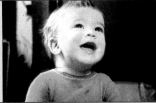 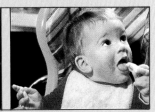

Stay sitting when placed

Turn when hears noise or call

Hold and feed himself with crust

12-20 MONTHS

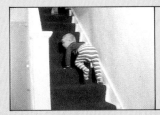 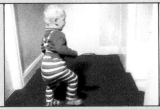 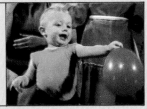

Go up and down stairs by himself

Toddle

Say 4 or 5 words

who are later than average in walking or talking or being dry may have a parent who had a similar pattern of development, whereas other slow developers are more cautious than most, and delay in standing or walking may simply be due to fear of falling, rather than lack of ability.

The illustrations on pages 38–9 show the times when babies usually start particular activities. If your baby is not performing all the activities shown by the last age in the range you should make sure he is seen by your doctor. He may still be a normal baby even if he has not attained the abilities by that age, but it is important to confirm this with medical advice.

When assessing his abilities remember that if your baby was born two months prematurely you need to subtract this length of time from his age to determine his developmental age. For example, when your two-months premature baby is three months old he should perform similar activities to a baby aged one month who was born at full term.

Communication

As we saw in Chapter 1, newborn infants can see and hear, and eye-to-eye contact between the mother and infant provides the first means of communication between them. Newborns respond to their mother's voice or the expressions on her face by blinking, facial expressions, movements of the limbs, drawing in breath or stopping feeding. Crying, of course, is another of the newborn's methods of communication.

A social smile, which is a copying of the mother's expression, usually first occurs at about the age of six weeks but often happens earlier. Gurgling noises usually come at about the same time. At three or four months your baby 'talks' in his own incomprehensible language if you talk to him; so, as I mentioned in the previous chapter, it is important that you talk to your baby from birth even though you may feel awkward doing so. The more you talk to your baby the earlier his communication abilities and speech will develop.

At about eight months he may make 'mm' and 'dada' sounds, although they do not have any meaning.

Three out of four children say one word with meaning by the age of twelve months and at about this time your child talks in his own language which nobody else can understand but which is more sophisticated than his meaningless burblings at four months. By about two years the average child puts two or three words together to make a phrase. In the second and third year indistinct speech is common, especially a lisp or stutter. It usually resolves by itself, provided you make no attempt to remedy it. If a stutter persists beyond this age and causes your child distress, you should mention it to your family doctor, or visit a properly qualified speech therapist. Special therapy for this problem is very often completely successful.

Delayed development   The meaning of words is usually understood by children long before they can say them. Speech development will be delayed if you do not talk to the child, but twins are often late in talking, perhaps because their mother has less time to talk to them or because they communicate with one another well enough without speech.

Delay in talking is never due to the fold of skin under the tongue being too tight. Though widely believed in, so-called 'tongue-tie' does not exist. Deafness, on the other hand, *will* cause speech delay. Deafness is often only partial, which can make it harder for you to recognize that there is a problem, but means that medical help can enable your child to hear sufficiently well for speech difficulties to be overcome. 'Serous otitis', which can result from ear infections, can also affect your infant's hearing and speech development (see Chapter 4). If you are worried that your child cannot hear normally at any age, you should arrange with your family doctor for his hearing to be checked as soon as possible.

Your child's development does not, of course, stop at two years of age, but if there are going to be any problems with development, they are nearly always apparent by this age.

Crying babies

The sounds of a baby's crying due to illness, pain and hunger have been scientifically analyzed and found to be different. But the differences are so subtle that most parents cannot distinguish between them. During the first few months infants do not shed tears when they cry, but this does not mean that they are pretending.

Crying is the only way your baby has for communicating his needs. In fact it is more likely that your baby is unwell if he is abnormally quiet or 'good'. But if your baby often cries persistently during the first weeks, he should be seen by your doctor, who will check for any physical cause. In most instances no physical ailment is found, and in nearly all cases the problem resolves by itself when the infant reaches about three months.

Persistent crying may be very wearing for both parents and be seemingly endless. Whether your baby cries a lot or not, it is helpful for both of you to take off one or two evenings each week to visit friends or go out for a meal or to a movie, as this will help to put problems into perspective.

Hunger and thirst
Babies often cry and become restless before a feed is due, and in the early weeks of life yours may demand to be fed every three hours or even every two hours. This is perfectly normal for a breast-fed baby, or even for a bottle-fed baby receiving modern milk preparations. Babies born early need particularly high volumes of milk to catch up the growth that should have occurred earlier. They may become less demanding when they have grown a little bigger.

Recommended volumes of milk for babies are only the average amounts, and many infants will need more to prevent hunger. Regular weighing and measuring, and the use of a growth chart to plot and check the results are the only ways of ensuring that your infant is receiving the correct amount of feed (see earlier in this chapter).

Feeding by the clock at regular intervals often leads to crying, and the modern practice, as I mentioned previously, is to feed your baby when he demands it.

A few infants scream when they are brought to the breast and this is often due to anxiety caused by previous failure to keep the infant's nose away from the breast during feeding. This feeling of smothering can be prevented by gently pressing down with two fingers on the top of your breast just above the brown area of the areola. This keeps your breast clear of your baby's nose, giving him room to breathe.

It is impossible to determine the difference between a cry due to hunger and a cry due to thirst. The only way of solving this problem is to offer your baby water twice daily. This can easily be given at the time when you normally take a midmorning and afternoon coffee break. Some babies dislike the taste of pure boiled water, so a little fruit juice or one level 5-ml teaspoonful of sugar can be added to 3 fl oz (100 ml) of boiled and cooled water – a lower concentration of sugar than is present in breast milk.

Colic

Colic usually begins at about two weeks of age and has usually stopped by four months. It is sometimes called three months' colic. The infant with colic screams, draws up his legs and cannot be comforted by feeding, being picked up or having his diapers changed. This screaming bout characteristically occurs in the early evening, when the mother is busy getting supper ready, has less time to play with her baby, and may be anxious. Breast-feeding mothers have less milk at that time of the day and this may be another factor.

Colic, though distressing and exhausting for baby and parents, is not a physical illness and does no harm to your baby. You should take your baby to the doctor if you suspect that he has colic, so that other causes can be ruled out. He or she may prescribe dicyclomine hydrochloride, an antispasmodic drug which might make your baby sleepy, and which seems to help in many cases of colic. This medicine is prescribed only for typical three months' colic which occurs in the evening and therefore only one dose of the medicine should be given per day until your baby is over his bouts of screaming.

Some pediatricians recommend giving small quantities of Chamomile tea, which can be soothing.

Feeding problems

It is widely thought that crying after a feed is due to over-feeding or the breast milk not agreeing with the baby. But these beliefs are in fact nothing more than old wives' tales. A far more likely cause is babies gulping down excessive air at the beginning of a feed and then having difficulty expelling it. This happens either because the milk spurts too plentifully from the breast, or because the hole in the bottle's nipple is too small. I have explained what you can do to help with these problems in Chapter 1.

Lack of physical contact

Even the newborn infant cries to obtain physical contact and he will stop as soon as you pick him up. You won't be spoiling your baby if you pick him up whenever he wants contact. Once he is a few weeks old and begins to be awake for longer periods, he may not tolerate being left alone in his carriage or crib, bawling every time you disappear from view. Putting your baby into a harness which allows him to remain in contact with your body while you move around will almost certainly keep him contented. Alternatively, you can lie him in a canvas 'bouncer' chair from as early as a month and place him in a safe position in the kitchen or wherever you are working (see page 18). He should not be so miserable once he can see you and be talked to.

If your baby does not stop crying when he is being held, try walking with him and rocking him in your arms or in his carriage, or taking him for a car ride. Or try the old swaddling method of wrapping him firmly in a blanket and putting him into a small cot. Although you are not giving him physical contact, being tightly tucked up gives many babies a cozy feeling of security which puts a stop to their crying.

Sucking the nipple without obtaining milk stops babies crying, provided they are not hungry. Putting a pacifier into your crying baby's mouth if he is not hungry may be effective as a temporary measure, and, like allowing him to suck purely for comfort on the nipple, this method is not psychologically harmful for your baby. At one time pacifiers were frowned upon by the medical profession, as it was thought that they caused deformity of the mouth, but provided that it is not in the mouth continuously and you use the more modern designs which are carefully shaped to fit the mouth, these complications will not occur.

Failure of mother-infant bonding

Crying may be a sign of difficulties between mother and baby. It is now considered by experts that this may be related to the character of the baby as much as the response of the mother. Crying may be the result of each having difficulty adjusting to the other. If your baby has been crying a lot of the time for several weeks you may become depressed, but alternatively the depression could be the cause of your infant's crying, as mothers have difficulty in responding lovingly to their babies when they are feeling fed up. If you are feeling thoroughly despondent and dejected it is best to seek your doctor's help, as depression can be treated effectively today. It is also a good idea to join a local postnatal support group where you can share your troubles with other mothers, many of whom will be going through the same problems as you. You can read more about this subject in *Anxiety and Depression* by Prof. Robert Priest, also in this series.

Special problems after three months

Loneliness is probably the most common cause of crying after the age of three months. While awake during the day your infant may not put up with being left alone but is happy if he is in the room where you are working. He is extremely interested in his surroundings and needs the stimulation of things going on around him to prevent him from becoming bored and lonely.

Separation from the mother during admission to the hospital or when parents go on vacation by themselves may be followed by bouts of crying. Your infant is only able to recognize about two or three adults at a time and frequent changes in the caretaker may be associated with crying.

Fear After about five months your baby may cry when a stranger approaches him or when he sleeps in a different room. He may wake suddenly, sobbing, and appear terrified, probably due to a nightmare, although there is no method of proving it. This sort of fearful behavior is quite normal for babies, and is no cause for concern. Nearly all grow out of it in time.

Other causes

Illness If your baby suddenly starts crying persistently, especially if he has not cried like this before, you should suspect that he is ill and call the doctor. Middle ear infection, know as otitis media (see Chapter 4), often causes persistent crying at night, and, rarely, meningitis (Chapter 3) or a urinary tract infection (Chapter 5) may have no signs other than crying.

If your baby cries when straining to have a bowel movement he may be constipated. In severe constipation the skin of the rectum may become cracked, causing intense pain. A visit to the doctor will be necessary to confirm the diagnosis and for treatment to be prescribed (see Chapter 5).

If your infant has sudden attacks of screaming and appears pale, and these attacks last for a few minutes and recur every ten to twenty minutes, he may have a serious intestinal problem such as intussusception (see Chapter 5) and you should make sure that he is seen by a doctor within an hour or two. If a doctor is not immediately available he should be taken to be seen at a hospital.

Teething   See page 47.

Changing   Babies do not seem distressed when their diapers are wet or soiled unless they have diaper rash (see Chapter 6), although some do cry and struggle when they are being undressed or changed. Diversionary tactics, such as singing a rhyme or dangling a rattle from your mouth, may be required to keep your baby calm enough for changing time not to become an ordeal for you both.

Tiredness   When your baby has been on a long journey or has been stimulated more than usual by playing with relatives, for example, he may become irritable, cry inconsolably and not be able to sleep. More than likely he will be back to his usual self by the next morning.

Sedation

In most babies who cry a lot none of the physical causes that have been described above are present. If your baby has been examined by a doctor and no physical cause for the problem has been found it is likely to resolve by itself.

However, if you are at the end of your rope he or she may recommend a short course of sedation for your baby with promethazine hydrochloride, a mild over-the-counter drug. This would only be for a week or so to enable you to regain some of your strength. But don't give this medicine for longer than your doctor suggests as it loses its effect and may make your baby irritable after that time.

Sleeping problems

In the first few weeks of life some babies sleep almost continuously throughout the twenty-four hours, whereas others sleep only about twelve hours. Many mothers consider that their newborn baby should sleep continuously and are not aware that he might be taking an interest in what is going on around him.

Few babies can manage without a night feed for the first few months. To help you get more sleep after the first three weeks, try to organize your baby's night feeds into a pattern that suits you. For example, feed him as you are going to bed so that you get the maximum amount of sleep before he wakes up for his next feed.

The age at which babies sleep through the night and do not require night feeds varies greatly. It will probably happen when your baby weighs about 11 lb (5 kg) and you should not worry if your neighbor's child of a similar age has already dropped his night feed and yours still demands it. But by five months of age most babies do not demand more than one feed during the night.

If your baby needs little sleep he may wake regularly at 2 or 4 am and remain awake for two or three hours. Sometimes you may be able to settle him with a drink but when this fails you may be tempted to take him into your own bed before he goes to sleep. In my opinion this is not a good idea because your baby may be reluctant to leave your bed later, and the routine then becomes a habit. Some babies wake very early but are then content to remain awake looking at mobiles above their cribs, or playing with toys left in the crib.

During the night babies often open their eyes, lift their heads and move their limbs. If they are not touched or disturbed they fall back to sleep again. If your baby's crib is next to your bed you will probably wake as a result of this moving, get out of bed and take a look at him. Your baby may see or hear you, this may wake him up completely and then he will cry. If your baby sleeps in a separate room you won't hear these movements, wake up and disturb him. If you are worried that you might not hear him if he becomes ill during the night in a separate room, you can install a cheap electronic baby alarm that will enable you to hear him without him hearing you.

There is no easy solution if your baby tends to wake in the middle of the night, refuses to go back to sleep and persists in crying. It may help to leave a small reading light on or leave the door open with the light from the hall shining into the room and to make sure that there are no frightening pictures or objects in the room. Mild sedatives such as promethazine hydrochloride given when your infant wakes may be effective for up to a week but as I have said before this drug often makes babies irritable in the morning. As your baby grows older he will become more able to amuse himself with his toys if he wakes up in the early hours, and by the age of two years he may well have changed his sleep pattern so that he wakes later at 6 am, which is more acceptable to you.

If you want your baby eventually to sleep in a separate room, it is best to move him out of your bedroom before the age of five or six months, as sleep disturbance caused by such a move is less likely to follow at that age.

Many parents have difficulty getting their baby off to sleep at night. Infants drop off more easily at this time if you set up a repeated bedtime ritual. A warm bath followed by being wrapped in a particular blanket may later be replaced by you or your partner reading from a book or singing nursery rhymes before the light is turned out. Even small infants may be upset and slow to settle if you change these routines. Soft, cuddly toys give a baby a reassuring sense of security while he's dropping off to sleep. You can put one in your baby's crib from shortly after birth.

Avoiding problems while weaning

Ideally you should gradually reduce breast-feeds over a period of several weeks after three solid meals daily have been introduced. Increasing amounts of solids can then be given to replace the calories lost by reducing the amount of milk. The first feed to omit is the midday feed, and then the early morning feed and finally the late-night feed.

You may find it difficult to reduce breast-feeding as your infant looks imploringly at the breast to try to persuade you to give him another feed. As with every other aspect of separation between mother and child this should be considered part of the process of your child growing up and having an independent existence. If your child seems miserable at the times of day he was accustomed to be breast-fed, a pacifier may help for a short period of the day to give the oral stimulation previously provided by the breast.

As mentioned previously, the occasional use of a pacifier does not affect the growth of the mouth and there are no medical objections to using them as long as they do not become a persistent habit. They should not be dipped in honey, though, or any other sweet fluid as this increases the risk of tooth decay.

The age at which you choose to stop breast-feeding is, of course, your own decision. Many babies nowadays are still being breast-fed at the age of six months, and some up to a year and beyond.

Teething

There is considerable variation in the age at which the first tooth is seen. It can appear at any time between six and twelve months, the first teeth usually being the lower incisors, that is, the middle teeth at the front of the lower jaw. The order in which the rest of the teeth emerge is shown in the diagram overleaf.

From the age of a few weeks babies normally put their fingers, and later anything else that comes to hand, into their mouths, and this has nothing to do with teething.

Teething produces only teeth. It does not, contrary to popular belief, cause fever, diarrhea, diaper rash or convulsions. So if your baby has any of these symptoms, don't pass them off as being due to teething; make sure he sees a doctor.

Some infants appear to have pain during the first day or so that the teeth are coming through the reddened gums. You will need to comfort your teething baby and distract him from the pain. A dose of acetaminophen syrup given by mouth usually stops this pain and if necessary the dose can be repeated after six hours. Biting on something hard seems to help the discomfort, so try giving your baby a cooled water-filled teething ring to bite on. Mild pain-relieving ointments are available but they are effective for only a short time because they are quickly washed away by the baby's saliva.

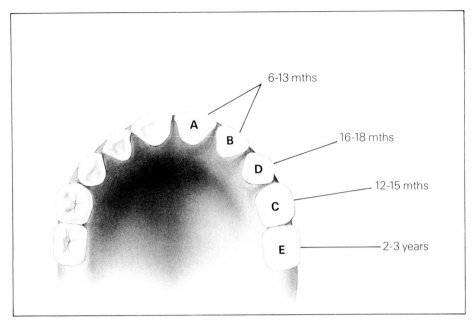

6-13 mths

A

B

16-18 mths

D

12-15 mths

C

2-3 years

E

You can see new teeth just protruding through your baby's gums. Babies will put their hands in their mouths well before teething begins.

If no tooth appears and yet he seems to be in pain for longer than six hours, it is possible that your baby is ill – perhaps with an ear or urinary tract infection (see Chapters 4 and 5) – and so your doctor should be consulted.

So far we have looked at the health problems that most often affect babies during the first months of life. In the next chapter I show how to recognize, prevent and treat the common infectious diseases, which can be caught by children of any age.

3. THE COMMON INFECTIOUS DISEASES OF CHILDHOOD

Infectious diseases are caught by every child. They are caused by germs – bacteria or, more commonly, viruses – invading the body and are passed on from one child to another, usually in minute droplets that are coughed or sneezed into the air by someone who has the disease. These germ-carrying droplets can carry for at least 10–15 ft (3–4.4 m). Most infectious diseases are caused by viruses. These are not affected by antibiotic drugs, so you have to wait for your child's own immune system to overcome the infection.

Until he is six months old, your baby has some immunity to many of the infectious diseases but not to whooping cough. This immunity is given by antibodies from the mother's blood that crossed the placenta into his bloodstream during pregnancy. Your infant's own antibodies can be produced by immunization (see later in this chapter).

The time between catching the infection and the symptoms first appearing is called the incubation period. This ranges from two days with scarlet fever to forty with infective hepatitis (see chart on page 66). With many of these diseases, the infected person can pass the infection on before the symptoms appear. So by the time you know your child has caught the illness, he will probably already have given it to members of the household who have not had the disease before or been immunized. There is no value, therefore, in enforcing a quarantine period during which your sick child is separated from the rest of the family. But while your child is still infectious (see chart on page 66) it would be wise not to let him come into contact with people from outside the family who have not had the disease before or who have not been immunized. It is rare to get one of the common infectious diseases twice.

If you suspect that your child is coming down with one of the common infectious fevers, do not take him to see the doctor, as your child could infect other people at the doctor's office. And in any case, unless there are complications, there may be no treatment your doctor can give. Telephone your doctor instead and he should be able to confirm the diagnosis and give advice on what to do.

Do your best for your child's health by having him immunized (see page

75), but there is no need to be overprotective, keeping him away from other children in case they are infectious. Some of these ailments, it is true, will make your child feverish and miserable for a while, which can be upsetting for you at the time. But you can be reassured that it is much better for your child to catch these diseases while young, rather than later in life when they can be much worse.

In this chapter I deal first with the infectious fevers themselves, such as measles and mumps; I then explain how to cope with your child's high fever and the possible complication of febrile convulsions; and finally I cover immunization.

The childhood fevers

Measles
This ailment makes children miserable. It is rare during the first six months of life if the mother had measles as a child, as her immunity is passed on to her baby.

The incubation period is ten to fifteen days and your child is infectious about six days before the rash appears and for five days afterwards. The measles virus is spread by minute droplets from the nose and throat of

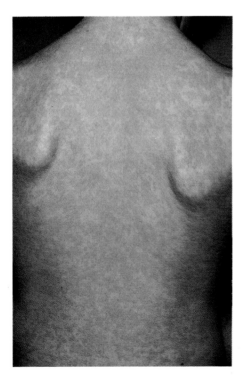

Measles rash after the third day of infection, covering the entire body.

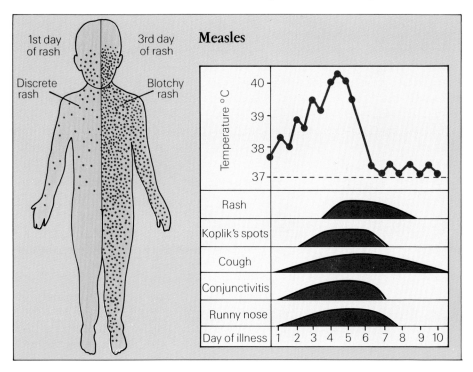

A symptom guide for measles, showing the characteristic changes in the development of the disease over 10 days.

infectious children and 90 per cent of family contacts are liable to catch the disease if they have not had it before or have not been immunized.

Symptoms The first symptoms are often a slight rise of temperature, a runny nose, redness of the eyes (conjunctivitis), lethargy and loss of appetite, together with a cough. A cough is essential for the diagnosis of measles. Although children with measles don't like bright light, it won't actually harm their eyes. If your child complains that the light is hurting his eyes, draw the curtains and reduce the light in his room for comfort.

Two or three days later white spots (called Koplik's spots), about the size of a pinhead, with a surrounding red area, can be seen on the inside of the cheeks close to the lower back teeth. The spots inside the cheeks only last a few days and are followed by the characteristic rash which appears in conjunction with a sharp rise in temperature (which may be as high as 104°F (40°C). The rash is red, slightly raised and rapidly becomes blotchy, but it is not itchy. It first appears behind the ears and on the face and spreads to the chest during the next twenty-four hours. Then it spreads to the arms and legs and reaches the feet by about the third or fourth day.

At this time the rash fades on your child's face and his temperature falls. By now he will be feeling much better and will begin to eat again.

Remember that several drugs, particularly penicillin, cause a rash very similar to that of measles. Also, other viruses such as those of German measles and mononucleosis produce a similar rash (see later in this chapter). All these should be suspected if the course of your child's illness is different from that described here.

As the rash fades there may be a mild fine peeling of the skin and occasionally there is brownish discolouration of the skin. These after-effects clear up within a few days.

Possible complications If any of the following occur you should inform your doctor.

Middle ear infection (see Chapter 4) is the commonest complication of measles, and symptoms, particularly waking with earache at night, usually occur about three days after the onset of the rash.

Occasionally a chest infection (bronchopneumonia, see page 92) occurs and this is shown by an increasing cough, a fast rate of breathing and sometimes by persistence of fever when the rash has gone.

Rarely the child's red eyes will become infected and will exude a yellowish discharge.

Very rarely encephalitis (inflammation of the brain) occurs but this only happens in about 1 in 500 children with measles and usually starts four to five days after the onset of the rash. The warning signs are increasing drowsiness, vomiting or irritability. If you notice any of these symptoms at this stage of the illness you should ask your doctor to see the child. Fortunately recovery from encephalitis is usually complete, with no lasting harm done to the brain.

Treatment and prevention No antibiotics have any effect on the virus which causes measles. Treat the fever as described on page 66. If your child's eyes become crusted, swab them gently with cotton wool dipped in cooled boiled water.

The complications of middle ear and chest infection are treated with antibiotics, but cannot be prevented by them. If there is discharge from the eyes, your doctor will prescribe an antibiotic eye ointment to clear up the infection (see page 20). The infection will not damage your child's eyesight.

Your child should be allowed to get up from bed as soon as he wants to.

Infants can be immunized against measles between the ages of twelve to fifteen months, depending on which country you live in (see page 72 and the chart on page 75). Most children who are not immunized will catch the disease.

German measles (Rubella)

This is usually a mild illness and causes few problems, except for the fetus if the mother catches German measles in pregnancy – especially in the first five months. The virus is different from the one that causes measles. Probably about one in four children who have contracted German measles have no rash but blood tests show that the disease has given them future immunity.

German measles is rare in the first six months of life if the mother has had the infection or has been immunized. The incubation period is ten to twenty-one days and the virus is spread by droplet infection from the nose or throat of an infected person. It is infectious a day before the rash appears and for two days after its appearance. About 50 per cent of brothers or sisters who have not had the disease before will be infected if they have not been immunized.

Symptoms   Your child may feel unwell for a day but in around three cases out of four the first sign of the illness is the rash which begins on the face, rapidly spreads to the trunk and lasts about three days. The spots are pink, pinpoint size, separate (not blotchy like measles), and are not raised above the normal level of the skin. They are not itchy. There is usually no fever but the rash may be accompanied by a slight runny nose and a little redness of the eyes, less severe than with measles. Several drugs may produce a similar rash and also other viruses, particularly those of roseola infantum (see page 55) and mononucleosis (see later in this chapter).

Frequently the glands in the neck swell up, particularly those at the back of the head and behind the ears. The glands in the armpits and groin may also be enlarged and possibly tender. They remain swollen for only a few days.

Possible complications   Encephalitis is extremely rare, affecting only about 1 in 5,000 children with German measles. It may precede the rash or occur during the week after it begins. If you notice the symptoms ask your doctor to see your child. Recovery is usually complete, with no lasting ill effects.

The main worry about German measles is the effect of the virus on the fetus during the first five months of pregnancy. It can cause abnormalities such as deafness, blindness and mental handicap. If any rash occurs during pregnancy see your doctor. He or she will take a blood test immediately and again ten days later to find out whether you have been recently infected with German measles. If the blood test is positive, your doctor will discuss the possibility of terminating the pregnancy. If a previous blood test has shown that you have had German measles before or have been immunized, no tests are needed, as the fetus is protected.

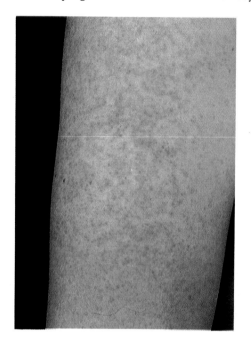

German measles rash after the third day of infection when the spots have moved from the trunk to the extremities of the body.

Below: A symptom guide for German measles, showing the slight rise in temperature.

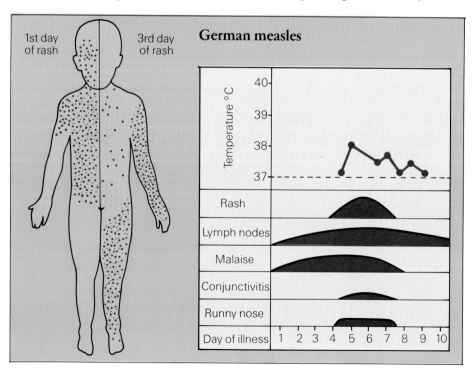

Treatment and prevention No treatment is necessary for German measles and you should not keep your child in bed. There is no method of preventing brothers and sisters from catching the illness if they have not had it before nor been immunized. See the chart on page 75 for immunization schedules in different countries. It is preferable to have your child immunized rather than to try to expose him to the disease while he's young, as complications are far less common with the vaccine than the natural disease virus.

Roseola infantum
This is a rarer disease than measles or German measles. The incubation period is seven to seventeen days and roseola occurs most commonly between the ages of six months and three years.

Symptoms Very high fever is a notorious feature of roseola infantum and is the first symptom. Your child's temperature will reach 102°–104°F (39°–40°C) and remain at this level for about three days. During this time he will be very irritable and refuse to eat. But he will play and behave

A symptom guide for Roseola, showing the notorious high fever during the first 4 days of infection.

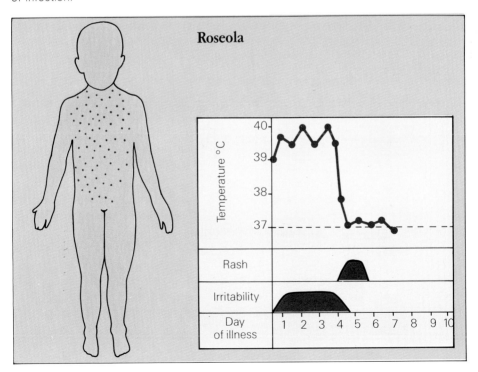

normally if his temperature is reduced by following the advice for coping with fever on page 66.

After three days his temperature will fall sharply and he will become less irritable. At the same time separate pink pinpoint spots will appear on his trunk. The rash is similar to German measles (see previously) and is not itchy. The spots rapidly spread to his limbs and face and completely disappear within twenty-four hours.

Possible complications   At the onset of roseola, as the temperature is rising rapidly, there is the slight risk of a febrile convulsion (see page 70). Also, the glands in the neck and at the back of the head as well as those behind the ears are often swollen during the illness, but return to normal once the infection is over.

Treatment   Apart from routine nursing to help lower the fever (see page 66) no other special treatment is needed. Although your child will not be keen to eat, he should be encouraged to take fluids (at least 20 fl oz/570 ml in twenty-four hours). Immunization against roseola is not available.

Chickenpox (Varicella)

This disease can occur at any age, including the newborn period. The incubation period is eleven to twenty-one days. Chickenpox is spread by droplet infection from the nose and throat. Your child is infectious from the day before the rash until about six days after it appears. The dry scabs do not contain active virus. About 75 per cent of other children in the home will catch the virus if they have not had chickenpox before. A second attack is very rare.

Symptoms   The spots appear in crops starting as raised pimples and changing to blisters within about twelve hours. Your child may have a fever, rising to a maximum of around 102°F (39°C) on the second day. During days two and three the fluid in the blisters becomes cloudy and dries, forming a scab. During the first three or four days of the illness new crops of pimples appear, especially on the trunk and later on the face and scalp. Urticaria, a common allergic rash, may be confused with chickenpox on the first day (see Chapter 6). Urticaria tends to recur and should be suspected if the rash appears more than once.

If there are spots in the mouth they produce painful shallow ulcers, and if they are in the breathing passages they produce a severe cough. The glands in the neck or under the armpits may be swollen and tender. The spots itch but you should discourage your child from scratching, as this may produce secondary infection and scars. Keep his fingernails short and clean to help prevent this.

Possible complications   About 1 in 10,000 children develop encephalitis (see page 52), usually about five days after the onset. If you suspect encephalitis call your doctor immediately. Complete recovery is usual.

Chickenpox may be caught from a patient with shingles, since the two diseases are caused by the same virus – varicella zoster. Shingles is due to reactivation of the virus which has remained dormant in nerves, sometimes for many years after an attack of chickenpox. Elderly people with shingles suffer pain in the area of the spots, which can be severe. (see chart on page 66).

Treatment and prevention   Treat the fever as described on page 69. Calamine lotion may reduce the itching, or your doctor might prescribe an antihistamine drug such as promethazine hydrochloride to alleviate this symptom. If the spots become infected and ooze pus, consult your doctor. He may prescribe antibiotics to treat this secondary bacterial infection.

There is no way of preventing brothers and sisters from catching the illness and immunization is not available at present, although, at the time of writing, a new vaccine is being studied in Japan and the United States.

Scarlet fever
This disease is caused by bacteria called streptococci.

Symptoms   After an incubation period of two to four days your child will get fever, headache and a sore throat. Pinpoint red spots appear on the skin which fade if you apply pressure to them. They can be seen on the trunk and neck, but especially around the neck, in the armpits and groin. Your child will be infectious for ten to twenty-one days after the rash first appears. A thick white coating on the tongue peels on the third day, leaving a strawberry appearance. The rash lasts a few days and is followed by peeling of the skin.

Possible complications   Forty years ago this illness was dreaded because it was sometimes followed by rheumatic fever or kidney disease. In the Western world these complications are now extremely rare, and are not seen in large children's departments in hospitals for periods of up to five years.

Treatment   A ten-day course of penicillin given by mouth removes the bacteria responsible and may prevent other children from being infected. It is not possible to immunize against scarlet fever.

Mumps
This ailment is caused by a virus and affects the parotid gland which produces saliva and is situated over the angle of the jaw in front of the ear

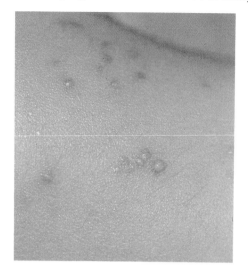

Chickenpox rash at an early stage, showing blisters.

Below: A symptom guide for chickenpox, showing the change in appearance of the spots as the disease progresses.

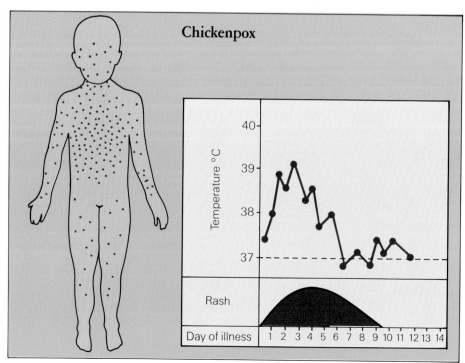

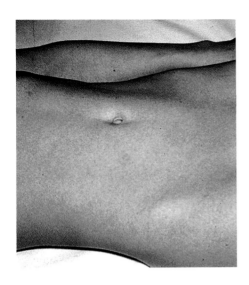

Scarlet fever rash within the first few days of infection.

Below: A symptom guide for scarlet fever.

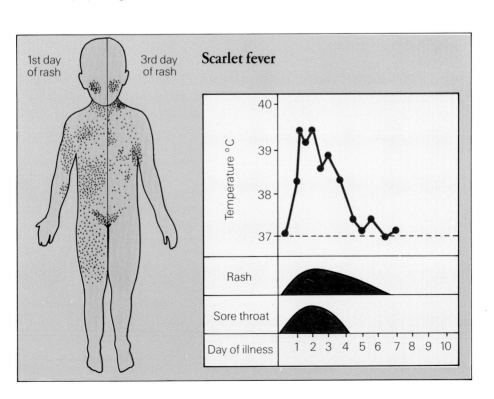

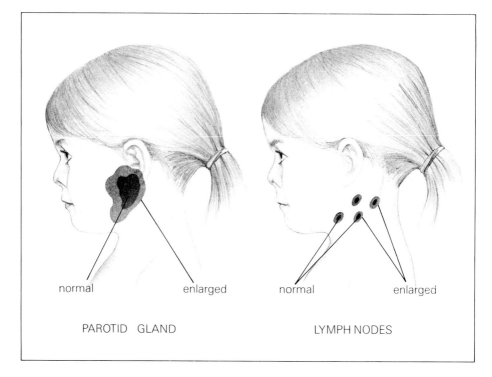

normal   enlarged   normal   enlarged

PAROTID   GLAND   LYMPH NODES

Mumps will cause painful swelling of the parotid glands and may be confused with swelling of the lymph nodes.

(see diagram above). It can affect the submandibular gland too, which also produces saliva and is located under the jaw. It rarely occurs in the first six months of life. If there is a swelling in these areas before the age of six months it is likely to be due to a large lymph gland infected as a result of tonsillitis (see Chapter 4).

The incubation period is twelve to twenty-one days. Mumps is spread by droplet infection and is infectious two days before the swelling appears until the swelling has gone. It is not very infectious, there being only a 1 in 5 chance that brothers and sisters in the household who have not had mumps before will contract it. By the age of fourteen years around 50 per cent of children have had an attack. Second attacks are rare.

Symptoms   The first symptom is usually pain and swelling in one or both parotid glands. The swelling makes the ear lobe move upwards and outwards, and reaches its maximum in about two days. It then subsides in about five days. The swelling becomes larger and more painful if your child eats or drinks something sour like lemon juice. Sometimes only one side of the face is affected. There is usually no fever.

Possible complications   The most worrying complication is inflammation of the testicles. Fortunately this is extremely rare before puberty. For this reason children with mumps should be kept away from men who have not had the disease.

Rarely inflammation of the pancreas occurs, causing abdominal pain three to four days after the glands near the jaw become swollen. Complete recovery follows without special treatment.

Encephalitis can occur even before the swelling of the glands and again recovery is complete (see page 52). If you suspect any of these complications, tell your doctor.

Treatment and prevention   Acetaminophen or aspirin may reduce discomfort, but your child does not need to stay in bed or have any other special treatment. Immunization against mumps is not carried out in Britain. It is given routinely in North America and Australia (see page 78 and chart on page 75).

Whooping cough (Pertussis)
This is one of the most serious of the common infectious diseases, and is caused by bacteria called Bordetella pertussis. The infection can occur at any age, the newborn infant receiving no protective immunity from his mother. The incubation period is seven to ten days and the germ is spread by droplet infection. If brothers and sisters are not immunized there is a 7 out of 10 chance of their contracting the disease. If they *are* immunized their chances of contracting the illness are reduced to 2 out of 10. Immunized children also seem to have a milder illness. A child will be infectious from about two days before the onset of the cough until about three weeks later. Contacts who have no symptoms for two weeks after exposure have usually escaped infection.

Symptoms   The illness can be divided into three stages and each lasts about two to three weeks:

1. The catarrhal stage
2. The paroxysmal stage
3. The convalescent stage.

Whooping cough is difficult to diagnose during the catarrhal stage, when there is a slight cough with sneezing which is often mistaken for an ordinary cold (see Chapter 4). The cough is particularly severe at night.

The paroxysmal stage starts with severe bouts of ten to twenty short dry coughs which occur both day and night, but particularly forcibly at night. A long attack of coughing is followed by a sharp intake of breath, which may produce the crowing sound or whoop. Some children, especially babies, never develop the whoop. During severe episodes of coughing your child may vomit. And during an attack he may become red or even blue in the face and sweat. The severe repeated cough is due to the fact that the mucus is very thick and your child finds it difficult to cough it up.

About two weeks later the vomiting stops and the cough gradually improves. This is the convalescent stage. The total duration of the cough is usually between two and three months and for this reason the Chinese call it the hundred-day cough. If your child has a cough which occurs in bouts, especially at night, and makes him vomit, the most likely diagnosis is whooping cough. Some children, though, have a milder attack and never vomit. If you suspect whooping cough, phone your doctor.

Possible complications   Occasionally partial blockage of one of the small tubes in the lung may occur as a result of obstruction by thick mucus. This happens most frequently in babies under six months of age and is shown by the infant being generally unwell, having a fever after the first week of the illness or having no improvement in the cough for four weeks after it has started. These symptoms would suggest bronchopneumonia. In

Gentle pats on the back will bring some relief to a child with whooping cough, but first take advice from a physiotherapist.

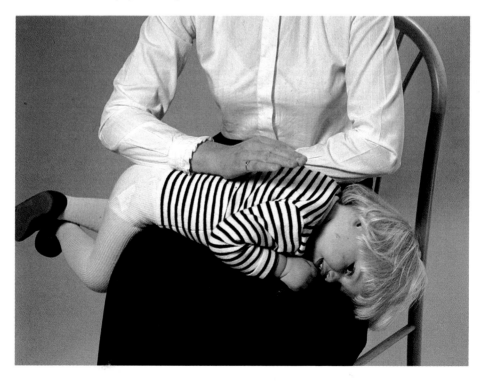

this case an X-ray of the chest will be taken to confirm the diagnosis. An antibiotic may be prescribed and physiotherapy to clear the blockage may help (see opposite).

In a severe episode the child may lose weight if he continues to vomit and is not given sufficient food. Crumbly food may trigger a coughing spasm that is forcible enough to cause vomiting. After this there is a short interval during which you can feed your child without provoking coughing.

Treatment for an established case of whooping cough is not very effective and is one of the strongest arguments in favour of immunization (see page 73).

If your doctor suspects whooping cough during the catarrhal stage (usually because a brother or sister has recently had whooping cough) he will prescribe a ten-day course of the antibiotic erythromycin for the affected child and any other children in the home. The antibiotic may shorten the course of the disease only if it is given in the early stages, but is unlikely to affect whooping cough once it is well established.

No medicine reliably improves the cough, but when your child's sleep is badly disturbed the barbiturate sedative, phenobarbitone might be prescribed, or large doses of promethazine, which is a milder drug.

Vomiting can be prevented in children by giving soft, non-crumbly food such as ice cream, or in babies by giving small amounts of fluid hourly.

In severe cases when the mucus is blocking one of the lung's small tubes you may be taught to give physiotherapy which helps to clear the secretions, especially before your infant goes to sleep. This consists of giving him a series of gentle pats on the back while he is lying down (see opposite). Ask the physiotherapist to teach you the right technique. An attack of coughing can be stopped by giving your child a gentle slap on the back while he is bent over your knee.

Babies under six months of age with whooping cough may need to be admitted to the hospital. This usually depends on discussion between parents and their family doctor. Rarely convulsions (see page 70) or coughing attacks severe enough to make your child turn blue due to lack of oxygen occur. These are both urgent reasons for children of any age to be admitted to the hospital.

Parents often become exhausted by sleep loss; arranging for different members of the family to sleep with the child will help to spread the load.

The cough usually lasts for eight to twelve weeks during the first episode but may recur when the child catches a common cold virus during the following year. Fortunately long-term effects on the lung are rare in developed countries.

Mononucleosis
Mononucleosis occurs most often in adolescents and young adults, but is not uncommon in children. Individual cases occur, although epidemics

may break out in schools. It is due to a virus which is found in the nose and throat. Close contact such as kissing is necessary for the disease to be passed on. The incubation period is known to be four to fourteen days, but as the duration of the illness is so variable it is not certain exactly how long the child with mononucleosis is infectious.

Symptoms start gradually after the incubation period. Poor appetite, fever and simply feeling ill are usually accompanied by a severe sore throat and enlarged glands in the neck, armpits or groin. The tonsils may be very painful and a thick white material may cover them. A blotchy red rash similar to measles (see previously in this chapter) appears in 10–20 per cent of mononucleosis sufferers. Your doctor may be able to confirm the diagnosis of mononucleosis with blood tests which are positive in about 60 per cent of patients during the first week of the illness but may become negative again within two to four weeks.

Possible complications   Jaundice – a yellowing of the skin and whites of the eyes – due to the mononucleosis virus affecting the liver can occur occasionally and resolves of its own accord within a few days. Other complications such as an infection of the lung or nerves are rare.

Treatment   There is no specific treatment for mononucleosis, but you can help reduce fever by following the advice on pages 66–72.

There may be a long period of feeling ill lasting up to several months. After being at home for a few weeks in the acute stage, it is important that your child returns to school as soon as possible once he feels a little better, preferably for half a day during the first week, as the depression which commonly follows this illness will be made worse if your child finds that he is falling behind with his school work. Going back to school early does not aggravate the physical condition and the risk of passing on the disease to schoolmates is slight.

There is no vaccine against mononucleosis.

Infectious hepatitis

This disease, which is an inflammation of the liver, is most commonly due to the hepatitis A virus. The number of hepatitis A cases has declined recently in developed areas of the world, although in southern Europe and in developing countries most people are infected by the time they reach adulthood.

Type A viral hepatitis has an incubation period of fifteen to forty days, the average being thirty days. The virus is spread from the feces and urine of an infected person.

Symptoms   Before the skin becomes yellow with jaundice there is often headache, nausea, vomiting, stomach ache and occasionally fever. As the jaundice increases, your child's appetite will improve. Your child's urine will be dark and the stools may be very pale. The jaundice lasts eight to eleven days, and your child is potentially infectious for no more than a week after the onset of jaundice.

Treatment and prevention   If your child wants to stay in bed he should be allowed to, although long bed rest is not essential. Fever can be controlled as described on pages 66–72. During the vomiting stage, you should give him small volumes of glucose mixture (see page 42) flavoured with fruit juice hourly during the day. As his appetite returns you can give him his usual diet, with no restriction on fatty foods. No drugs are needed. This condition is one of the mildest childhood infections and the outlook is excellent. But if drowsiness or jaundice last longer than two weeks your child should be seen again by the doctor.

If someone in your family has this type of hepatitis you can help prevent it spreading by scrupulous handwashing and by sterilizing food utensils, which is best done by boiling them for at least a minute. Also, your doctor might give other members of the family a preventive shot of human gammaglobulin, an extract from blood containing protective factors. This only helps if administered within the incubation period, and preferably within fifteen days of contact.

Meningitis

This disease is an inflammation of the membrane surrounding the brain and spinal cord called the meninges. It is uncommon, but most often affects infants between the age of six months and a year. It is usually caused by bacteria passing from the throat into the bloodstream, but can be due to a virus.

Symptoms   In children under three years it is difficult to recognize early signs of meningitis. The characteristic signs are refusal of feeds, drowsiness and convulsions (see page 70), but in the early stages there may just be fever, vomiting, irritability and a high-pitched cry.

Older children may have fever, vomiting and severe headache, but irritability, and particularly drowsiness or unusual behaviour, are the most distinctive features of this disease. Children with meningitis may also develop a dislike of bright light and have a stiff neck, which can be detected if you ask your child to look at his shoes. He will find this difficult to do. If he has spots which do not fade when you press them, this suggests that he may have a particular type of bacterial meningitis called meningococcal infection.

Treatment   Because the possible complications of meningitis are serious and include deafness and epilepsy, it is essential to act quickly if you suspect your child has the disease. You should consult a doctor within an hour. Urgent admission to hospital is needed for a lumbar puncture. In this procedure, which is carried out under a local anaesthetic, a needle is passed between the spinal bones in the lower part of the back to obtain a specimen of the fluid which bathes the spinal cord. This fluid is examined in the laboratory for signs of meningitis. If there is evidence of a bacterial infection, treatment is by antibiotics given by infusion into a vein. If this treatment is begun soon enough, your child will begin a full recovery after a few days. Meningitis caused by a virus usually clears up within a few days without special treatment.

Infectious diseases of childhood

Disease	Incubation period (days)	Infectivity
Measles	10–15	Six days before rash to five days after rash appears.
German measles	10–21	One day before rash to two days after rash appears.
Roseola infantum	7–17	Not known.
Chickenpox	11–21	One day before onset of rash until six days after first crop of spots started.
Scarlet fever	2–4	Ten to twenty-one days after onset of rash.
Mumps	12–21	Two days before swelling appears until swelling has gone.
Whooping cough	7–10	Two days before onset of cough until three weeks later.
Mononucleosis	4–14	Uncertain.
Hepatitis (A virus)	15–40 (average 30)	Up to one week after onset.

Coping with fever

Fever indicates that your child has an infection, and is often present in the few days before an infectious disease such as measles is confirmed by the spots. Fever may produce headache and redness of the skin and make your child irritable. He will probably want to drink much more than usual to replace the body fluids lost in sweating.

If your child has fever you should always let your doctor know if it is over 102°F (39°C). It is particularly important to inform him about any degree of fever if your infant is under six months of age.

Fever is the common feature of all the infectious diseases described in this chapter, but it accompanies several other common childhood ailments which I cover in other chapters, including:

- Acute ear infections (see Chapter 4)
- Tonsillitis (see Chapter 4)
- Other respiratory tract infections (see Chapter 4)
- Urinary tract infection (see Chapter 5).

Taking the temperature

The normal skin (taken in the armpit) and mouth temperature is 98.6°F (37°C). The normal temperature in the rectum is 99.5°F (37.5°C). If your child's temperature is 1°F (0.5°C) above these levels he has a fever.

You can take his temperature by using either a thermometer or the recently introduced temperature indicator strip. A clinical thermometer is more accurate, but an indicator strip is quicker and easier to use. Whichever method you use, don't take your child's temperature immediately after a bath, or a hot drink or meal, as you may get a falsely high reading.

The thermometer is a narrow glass tube with a bulb filled with mercury at one end and a temperature scale marked on the glass. The mercury is heated by the body, expands and rises up to a point on the scale which can be read.

Before taking your child's temperature make sure that the mercury is well below the normal mark, shown on the scale by an arrow. To get the mercury level down, hold the thermometer by the opposite end to the bulb and give it several sharp flicks of the wrist in a downwards direction. If your child is under the age of five, place the bulb of the thermometer under his armpit, making sure his arm is held close to his side. If over five years old, slip the thermometer under his tongue and tell him to close his mouth gently without biting on the thermometer. Never leave your child unsupervised with a thermometer in his mouth. After three minutes remove the thermometer and note the temperature. Then sterilize the thermometer by placing it in an antiseptic solution for a few minutes.

The temperature indicator strip is easier to use than the thermometer, especially with babies and toddlers, as it only needs to be placed against your child's forehead for one minute. The appropriate panel of the strip glows to show you the temperature. This method is not as reliable as a thermometer, so if in doubt check your infant's temperature with a thermometer (see photographs overleaf).

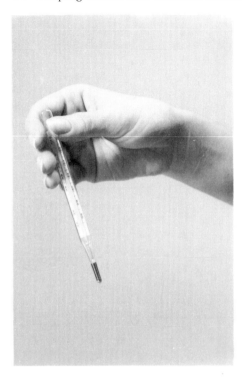

1. Flick the thermometer sharply to bring the mercury level down.

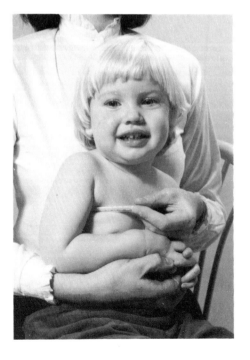

2. If your child is under five years of age, place the thermometer under the armpit for three minutes.

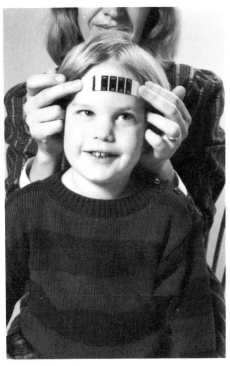

You will find it easier to use a temperature indicator strip for babies and toddlers.

What to do

Fever itself is not dangerous, but it may cause a convulsion if your child's temperature rises rapidly (see overleaf). The following tips should be useful in helping to prevent a rapid rise in temperature, in making your child more comfortable, and in helping you to cope more effectively with his fever:

- Acetaminophen can be given every six hours in recommended doses to reduce fever due to any cause.
- Don't wrap up your feverish child or take him into your bed, as this will only help his temperature to rise more rapidly.
- Taking off all your child's clothes and covering him with only a sheet may help.
- Ensure that his room is not hot and stuffy. In winter turn off the central heating, and in summer leave his window open. An electric fan is useful in hot weather.
- If he has a high fever, over 102°F (39°C), a few minutes tepid sponging at two-hour intervals may make him more comfortable.
- There is no need to confine your child to bed with a fever unless he is tired or in pain.

- It is perfectly safe to take your feverish baby or child in the open air to see your doctor. In fact, cool air may reduce his temperature and make it easier for your doctor to make the correct diagnosis.
- If your child is not keen to eat solid food you should encourage him to take fluids, and he can have any type he likes. A child of six months should be encouraged to have between 1–2 pt (500–1,000 ml) of fluid in twenty-four hours.
- There is no evidence to support the old saying, 'feed a cold and starve a fever.' If your child has fever you should neither encourage nor discourage him from eating solids. The main thing, as I have said, is to make sure that he drinks enough fluids.

Febrile convulsions

A convulsion is the only important consequence of fever. One child in thirty has a febrile convulsion between the ages of nine months and five years. To see your child suddenly go into a convulsion is a distressing and

Try to make your feverish child as cool and comfortable as possible.

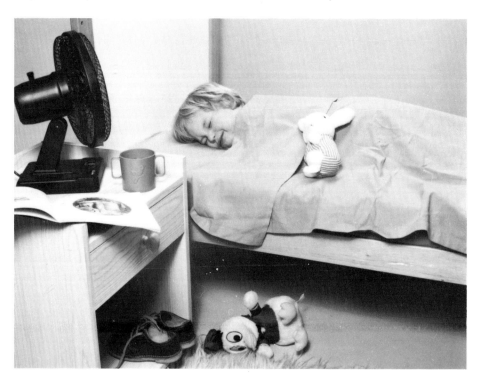

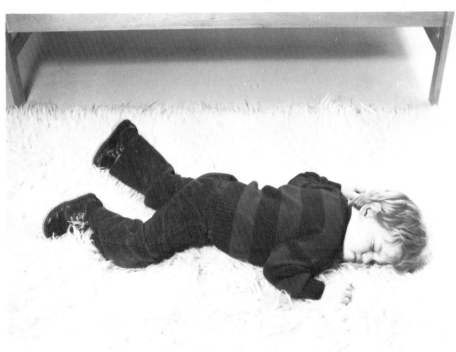

The emergency recovery position during a febrile convulsion.

worrying experience. Many parents have told me that at the time they thought their child was dying. It should be reassuring to know that most convulsions associated with fever last less than fifteen minutes, have absolu tely no lasting effect on your child and do not recur after the age of five years. These short convulsions do not affect your child's development.

Often fever is noticed only when a convulsion has already occurred. If your child has a seizure without fever your doctor will consider the poss- ibility of epilepsy.

A convulsion starts with a cry and loss of consciousness followed by rigidity of the whole body which lasts about half a minute. Finally there are jerking movements of the limbs or face.

Emergency treatment Remove all your child's clothes and cover him with a sheet only. Place him on his side or on his abdomen supported by a pillow, with his head to one side, to prevent him breathing vomit into his lungs if he is sick and to prevent his tongue from blocking his windpipe and choking him (see photograph above).

To cool him down try sponging him with cool water, applying a wet sheet to his trunk or putting him into a tepid bath. It is important to use tepid water rather than cold as the latter will close up the blood vessels in his skin and reduce the amount of heat loss. The ideal temperature is around 70°F (21°C), which is comfortable to the touch.

Never give fluids or medicines to your child if he is having a seizure or is semiconscious.

You should phone your doctor as soon as possible, or if he is not available immediately take your child to the nearest accident and emergency department of a hospital. On the journey he should be covered with a sheet or left undressed with underpants only; if he is covered up too much his temperature may rise and lead to a repeat convulsion. Cooling him by having no clothes on is the best treatment and cannot do him any harm.

Children who have a first convulsion usually need a short stay in the hospital. In most cases the high fever is due to a viral infection. When you reach the hospital your child may be given a shot to stop the seizure if it is still occurring. Most doctors give an additional shot of the anticonvulsant drug phenobarbitone to prevent a further attack occurring within a day or two. Your child may be given a lumbar puncture under local anaesthetic to exclude meningitis (see page 65).

Long-term outlook   About a third of children who had have a febrile convulsion will have further attacks which usually stop by the age of five years. If your child has already had a febrile convulsion you should follow carefully the advice given previously for controlling fever, especially the tips for keeping him cool. If your child has more than two episodes of febrile convulsions, a two-year course of anticonvulsant drug therapy may be considered. This won't affect the long-term outlook, but will reduce the chances of his having another seizure and of another harrowing experience for you.

Usually the decision about drug treatment is taken jointly between doctor and parents. A small percentage of children have an unusual type of convulsion – either affecting only one side of the body or lasting more than half an hour. This is another instance where the doctor may decide to prescribe anticonvulsant drug treatment for a period of two years to prevent recurrence of attacks.

Immunization

Immunity to several of the infectious diseases can be provided by the injection of vaccines. These are preparations of the germ causing the disease in which the germ is either killed or has been modified in the laboratory so that it causes a mild and usually undetectable infection. Your child's immune system is stimulated into producing antibodies specific to each disease, which give protection for many years, and in some instances for life. Immunization may protect your child alone (as in the case of tetanus) or it may reduce the chances of a younger and more susceptible member of your family catching the illness (as in whooping cough).

A great deal of adverse publicity about immunization has made parents worry whether they should allow their children to be immunized. It is important to understand that the controversy in Britain is about immunization against whooping cough only and that immunization with all the other vaccines currently used (except mumps, see page 78) is advised and accepted by all medical authorities throughout the world.

Whooping cough

Immunization against whooping cough is carried out during your baby's first year in three stages, the timing of each shot differing slightly from country to country (see chart on page 75). Research carried out in 1983 at the hospital where I work in London showed that the first shot gives your baby some protection against whooping cough; the second gives considerably more; and the third is a precautionary measure which may or may not confer extra protection. It is important, though, that your infant receives all three shots to maximize his chances of avoiding the disease. If for any reason, such as illness, your child does not receive his second or third shots at the recommended time, they will be just as effective if given later – even up to two years later. So don't worry if these shots are delayed; there is no need to start the whole course again.

Why should your child be immunized?   The main reasons why immunization against whooping cough is advisable are:

1. In North America children must be immunized before they go to school, and as a result whooping cough has virtually been eliminated here.
2. There is no effective treatment for whooping cough. Antibiotics such as erythromycin reduce the period your child is infectious but usually have no effect on the disease once it has begun. Cough medicines are also ineffective.
3. The vaccine reduces a child's chances of being infected by a member of the family who has whooping cough. As I pointed out earlier, two out of ten vaccinated brothers and sisters will contract the disease compared with seven out of ten unvaccinated brothers and sisters.

4. If children who have been immunized catch whooping cough they seem to have a milder and less distressing form of the illness.

Will there be any adverse reactions to immunization? The following reactions may occur following whooping cough vaccine:

1. It is not uncommon for your infant to be irritable and to have a slight fever a few hours after the shot, but this rarely lasts more than twenty-four hours.
2. Quite often there is redness and swelling at the site of the shot.
3. Often a small, hard lump which is not tender is found at the site of the shot and this may remain for several months. It is due to a small bruise and is no cause for concern.
4. Very rarely vaccination is followed by a high fever with convulsions and it is usually impossible to determine whether the fever was related to the immunization or was coincidental. These short convulsions do not cause brain damage (see page 70).
5. Brain damage, caused by encephalitis, is the complication that caused the recent controversy in Britain. If severe encephalitis occurs, it will do so within one week after the shot. It differs from a convulsion in that your child will become very drowsy and will vomit, rather than just having a temperature and convulsions. A recent study in Britain showed that normal children undergoing a full course of whooping cough immunization have a risk of about 1 in 100,000 of suffering permanent brain damage. This is the highest possible risk, and in fact it may be lower, as illness causing the encephalitis may occur coincidentally at the same time as the immunization. It may be reassuring to compare this risk with those of dying from the following:

- All accidents: 1 in 2,000
- Traffic accidents: 1 in 8,000
- Leukemia: 1 in 20,000
- Drowning: 1 in 30,000
- Travelling 500 miles (800 km) in a car: 1 in 100,000.

Opposite: A table of immunization schedules for Great Britain, United States of America, Canada and Australia.

VACCINE	Age in each country (up to 10 years)			
	UK	USA	Canada	Australia
Diptheria-tetanus-pertussis (DTP) + Polio (oral) (pertussis = whooping cough)	3 months 5 months 9 months 4½ years (pre-school)	2 months 4 months 6 months 4 years (pre-school)	2 months 4 months 6 months 4-6 years (pre-school)	2 months 4 months 6 months 5 years (pre-school)
Measles M **Measles–Mumps** MM **Measles–Mumps–Rubella** MMR	M–15 months	MMR–1 year	MMR–1 year	MM–1 year
Rubella (girls only)	10–13 years			10–14 years
B.C.G. (bacille Calmette-Guérin) against TB	10–13 years*			
Tuberculin test vaccine for TB		1 year		
Notes	*Best given at least 3 weeks before rubella. The age for B.C.G. varies with district.			

The risk attached to whooping cough immunization cannot be measured precisely but it really does appear to be extremely small. For example, recent research has revealed that no brain damage occurred after 80,000 whooping cough immunizations in North London, or after 180,000 immunizations in Glasgow, Scotland.

When should your child not be immunized?   Your infant should *not* be immunized against whooping cough if:

1. He has had previous seizures.
2. He had a local or general reaction to an earlier dose of whooping cough vaccine.
3. He has any acute infection, including a common cold. This applies especially at the beginning of the infection and when there is fever.
4. He was excessively irritable while severely ill during the first month of life.

Some areas are still controversial and in addition your doctor may decide not to immunize if:

1. You or your spouse, or your other children have had seizures.
2. Your child's development is delayed (see Chapter 2), or he has a disease affecting the brain, such as cerebral palsy.

Contrary to popular belief, if your child or one of his close relatives has asthma, hay fever or eczema, this is *not* a reason for avoiding immunization.

Measles
As I mentioned earlier in this chapter, measles is a miserable illness and its complications include middle ear infection, bronchopneumonia and encephalitis. Immunization provides protection in about 80 per cent of the children who receive the vaccine and the immunity lasts at least ten years.

It is given in one shot between the ages of twelve and fifteen months, depending on which country you live in (see chart on page 75). If it is given earlier, immunity is not so effective. If a healthy child who has not been immunized is in contact with a child with measles, protection against the disease can be provided by giving vaccine within three days of exposure.

In the past, measles was often diagnosed mistakenly and children denied the vaccine when they were not in fact protected. A dose of vaccine in children who have already had measles is not harmful.

Possible side-effects   Five to ten per cent of children have mild fever six to twelve days after the shot, which lasts twenty-four to forty-eight hours. Rarely there is a mild rash on the chest similar to measles (see previously in this chapter). One in five hundred children has a convulsion associated with this rise in temperature but this should be compared with the convulsion associated with fever which occurs once in every 150 children who have measles.

About one in ten thousand to one in a million infants develops encephalitis as a result of the immunization; but this should be weighed against the one in five hundred who develops encephalitis with measles.

When not to immunize   Measles vaccine should not be given if your infant has fever, is very undernourished, is receiving steroid drugs (for kidney disease, for instance) or has impaired resistance to infections due to a known long-term disease such as leukemia.

Infants who have had convulsions in the past or who are severely undernourished should receive measles vaccine only with an additional shot of low-dose human gammaglobulin into the other arm. Gammaglobulin is an extract from the liquid part of the blood which contains protective factors and reduces the possibility of mild fever developing in response to the measles vaccine.

If a child with long-term illness, such as heart disease, is not immunized and comes into contact with a child who has measles, a shot of gammaglobulin can be given which will prevent illness developing after this contact, but the protection will only last a few weeks.

German measles (Rubella)

All girls should be immunized against German measles to prevent them from catching the illness when they are pregnant, as this infection may have serious effects on the fetus (see previously in this chapter). In Britain and Australia the immunization is given at the age of ten to fourteen years and a blood test can be taken to find out whether the girl has previously had the infection. In North America the vaccine is given in a combined measles, mumps and rubella preparation at around twelve to fifteen months (see chart on page 75).

Immunization should be postponed if your child has fever, is receiving steroid drugs by mouth (for kidney disease, for example) or has impaired resistance to infections caused by a long-term disease such as leukemia. The vaccine may be effective for ten years or longer.

Rarely there is mild fever or rash about ten days after the shot, occasionally with enlargement of the glands in the groin and armpits, and pains in the joints. One child in half a million develops encephalitis after the shot, but one in five thousand develops it after German measles. Encephalitis following a shot of German measles vaccine does not result in brain damage.

Mumps

As mentioned above, North American children are immunized at around twelve to fifteen months of age with a vaccine containing mumps, measles and German measles vaccines simultaneously. This vaccine is not used in Britain and Australia, where mumps is not considered by the medical authorities to be a serious enough illness for immunization.

The mumps vaccine gives protection for at least twelve years, but protection for adult life given by having had the infection in childhood lasts much longer. Allergic reactions such as a rash are the only possible side-effects of the vaccine and these occur rarely and are mild. The reasons why the doctor might not give your child this vaccine are the same as for measles (see previously in this section).

Diphtheria

This is a dangerous throat infection which is now very rare in developed countries, thanks to mass immunization. But it is still common in many less developed countries and could be contracted during a vacation abroad. It is very important that all infants are immunized against this disease to prevent its recurrence in the future.

The vaccine is included in the triple vaccine which contains whooping cough, diphtheria and tetanus vaccines and is given in a course of three shots, the schedule depending on which country you live in (see chart on page 75). There are no reasons why your child should not receive diphtheria vaccine during the first five years of life, as it has no known side-effects. Immunity to diphtheria given by the vaccine lasts for life.

Tetanus

This is a dangerous disease affecting the nervous system, which is caused by a poisonous microorganism found in soil, dust and the excreta of grass-eating animals such as cows and horses. The classic symptom is lock-jaw. Fortunately tetanus is now very rare in developed countries, again largely due to mass immunization. It is essential that all children should be immunized, as a toddler can easily pick up tetanus from a dirty wound, and without the vaccine's immunity the mortality rate is high. The vaccine is included in the triple-vaccine shots (see chart on page 75 for immunization schedules). Immunity given by the vaccine lasts for ten years at least.

If your child has been immunized and has a dirty wound he should be seen by a doctor. The action he or she will take depends on the interval between the last tetanus shot and the injury. If the last immunization was received more than five years previously, your doctor will give one booster dose of tetanus vaccine. It is now considered inadvisable to give more booster doses than necessary, as the greater the number of doses the more possibility there is of provoking an allergic skin reaction. If the wound is severely contaminated with soil your doctor may give shots of penicillin as well as a preparation made from blood which contains protective factors against tetanus.

If your child has not been immunized he may be given an injection of the protective blood preparation and be started on a course of tetanus vaccine. If the wound contains soil, is dirty or deep he may also be given an antibiotic such as penicillin.

Polio

Poliomyelitis, to give the condition its full medical name, is a paralyzing disease which affects the limbs and the muscles, including those involved in breathing. It is caused by a viral infection but is now rare in developed countries thanks to immunization. It is still common in the Middle East and in Third World countries and so may be contracted while on vacation. All children should be immunized. It is given at the same time as the triple vaccine for diphtheria, tetanus and whooping cough. In Britain and Australia, it is given in the form of drops which are placed on the tongue (Sabin-type vaccine), while in North America it may also be given by shots (Salk-type vaccine). See chart on page 75 for immunization schedules.

Immunization should be postponed if your child has diarrhea, fever, is receiving steroid drugs by mouth, or has impaired resistance to infections due to a long-term disease such as leukemia.

Tuberculosis (TB)

TB is now so rare that many developed countries, such as the United States, Canada and Australia, do not include vaccination against the disease as a standard procedure in their nationally recommended schedules (see page 75). The BCG vaccine is given in certain parts of Britain where there is a higher rate of tuberculosis and for those travelling to Africa or Asia. It is not given if a child has eczema (see page 120) or impaired resistance to infection.

All immunized children develop a scab but about 1 in 200 children develops a shallow ulcer with discharge where the shot has been given; and the glands in the armpit may swell. These side-effects heal without treatment within about four months.

Flu

Immunization against influenza is advisable for children with long-term lung or heart disease but not for healthy children. Two shots a month apart are given initially, with a booster each year. The type of vaccine chosen will be the most effective one against the next type of expected flu epidemic.

Going abroad

Before travelling to a Third World country or to certain countries in southern Europe ask your doctor about special immunization shots, for yourself as well as your child. Depending on where you are travelling, he or she may immunize you against one or more of the following diseases:

- Typhoid fever
- Infectious hepatitis
- Cholera
- Yellow fever.

4. RESPIRATORY TRACT AND EYE PROBLEMS

In the previous chapter we looked at what are termed the infectious fevers, most of which have a generalized effect on your child's body. In the next two chapters I cover the common childhood ailments that affect particular areas of the body. This chapter is concerned with the top half of the body, namely with problems that affect the ears, nose, throat, chest and eyes; while Chapter 5 deals with illnesses of the bottom half: stomach troubles, genital problems and urinary tract infection.

Respiratory tract ailments

The respiratory tract consists of:

1. The upper respiratory tract, which comprises the ears, nose and throat.
2. The middle respiratory tract, comprising the larynx or voice box.
3. The lower respiratory tract, comprising the lungs, with their large and smaller tubes which distribute the air evenly to all parts of the organ.

Problems with the upper respiratory tract during childhood include the common cold, tonsillitis and ear infections; croup and inflammation of the epiglottis affect the middle respiratory tract; and bronchitis, bronchiolitis and pneumonia are infections of the lower respiratory tract. All of these ailments are covered in this section.

Viruses cause the greatest number of respiratory tract infections and are always responsible for colds, croup and bronchiolitis. At present there are no generally available effective drugs like antibiotics to treat them. On the other hand, all the infections listed above, except for colds, croup and bronchiolitis, can be due to bacteria. These are larger germs than viruses, which can be destroyed by antibiotics. The problem for treatment is that the same set of symptoms, say for example earache, may be due to any one of a large variety of viruses or bacteria. Your doctor will use his judgement as to whether your child's infection is due to bacteria or not, and depending on the severity of your child's condition will decide whether or not to prescribe an antibiotic.

Your doctor may take a throat swab which will be sent to a laboratory

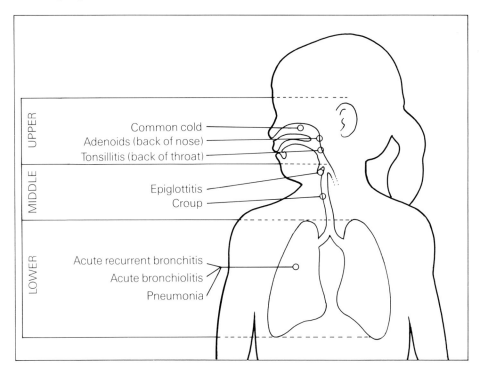

The common infections of the upper, middle and lower respiratory tract.

to find out whether bacteria or viruses are responsible for the infection, and, if the bacteria are the culprits, to determine their sensitivity to different types of antibiotics. For bacteria this process usually takes about forty-eight hours but it may take several weeks to obtain a viral result and your child will probably have recovered by the time it arrives. For this reason swabs are not usually taken, except for research purposes. So don't think your doctor is not doing his job properly if he doesn't take a throat swab.

Another difficulty is that some strains of bacteria are resistant to a particular antibiotic and this may only become apparent if your child fails to respond to a course of treatment. Thus if your child does not improve after a course of antibiotics the reason may be either that the infection was in fact viral, or that the bacteria were resistant to the antibiotic he was given. If this happens, or, as rarely occurs, your child's condition gets worse, you should of course inform your doctor, and he may then organize tests. The encouraging things to remember, though, are that the over-whelming majority of childhood respiratory tract infections clear up of their own accord, leaving no ill effects, and that all these infections become much less common after the age of seven to eight years.

The common cold

Infants and children have an average of about six colds every year, each caused by a different type of cold virus and not, as is popularly thought, by washing the hair or going out in the cold. As most of these occur in the winter your child may catch a new infection every three weeks. Infants in the first year of life may catch an infection from you or your spouse but they often have less severe symptoms than you. While your baby is breast-feeding he is likely to catch fewer colds than average.

Symptoms   A cold is often preceded by a sore throat. When it arrives the main symptoms are sneezing, mucous discharge from the nose and, rarely, fever. If your baby has a very runny nose he may find it hard to breathe while feeding, and sometimes this makes it impossible for him to feed at all. If so, you should see your doctor, who may be able to help your baby to feed normally again by giving salt solution nose drops.

The nasal discharge pours out of the nose or may go backwards over the tongue and make your infant cough. In young children the throat, ears and lungs are very close together and the infection in the nose may spread to the ears, causing earache (see overleaf), or to the lungs, causing coughing (see page 91), particularly at night when your child's position in bed helps the mucus to run back down his throat.

A single cold can last from three days up to three weeks, so there's no need to worry if it goes on for that long. Sometimes it can seem as if your child is never free of colds. This is because he is catching one cold after another in quick succession. If you watch his condition closely you should notice short symptom-free gaps between infections, indicating that there is no other underlying ailment such as asthma to worry about (see later in this chapter). Unless your child has a temperature over 102°F (39°C), has earache or has had his cold continuously for three weeks there is no need to see your doctor.

Treatment   There is no effective treatment for the common cold, and there is no need to keep your child in bed or indoors. In fact cool air helps to dry up the nasal discharge. If he is feverish, you can help to control his temperature by following the advice on pages 66–70. Your doctor won't prescribe antibiotics as they don't affect cold viruses. I do not recommend using decongestant nose drops, as there is a danger that they will run back down into the lower respiratory tract, carrying the infection into the lungs.

Many parents try to prevent their infants and children from getting colds by painstakingly avoiding contact with people who have cold symptoms. This approach is not advisable, for three reasons. First, it doesn't usually work, because colds are spread by droplet infection which carries for several feet from the infectious person; this means that you can catch a cold from a passerby in the supermarket, for example. Second, children have to experience infections such as colds in order to build up a degree of resistance for the future. And finally, if your child is susceptible to a bout of recurrent infections of this type he is bound to succumb to them at some stage in his life. Far better to get them over with early, before they have a chance of disrupting his school routine.

Earaches

These are very common in childhood. If your child is in the one- to four-year-old age group, you can expect him to have an earache two to three times a year. They often follow a cold or tonsillitis (see later in this chapter).

Symptoms   Earache is the main symptom of an ear infection, or otitis media, as it is known medically. If the middle ear is infected, secretions accumulate, producing an increase in pressure in the middle ear and this causes severe pain. Otitis media is one of the few causes of a fretful infant crying all night (see Chapter 2).

If your baby is under a year old it is often difficult to tell whether his discomfort is due to an ear infection as he may just keep crying. An older baby with earache may pull one ear, have a fever or vomit. Pulling gently on his ear lobes is not a good way to check whether he has earache, as this may not cause him pain even if he has an ear infection. To confuse the issue further, if your baby pulls at his ears it doesn't necessarily mean that he has otitis media. If your baby is miserable and/or feverish for no apparent reason, he should be seen by a doctor, as should any child who is suspected of having earache.

Infants and children usually dislike having their ears examined by a doctor, especially if they are painful. Your child will be less upset if he sits on your knee and you hold first one side of his head and then the other against your chest (see photograph opposite).

Possible complications   In a few children mucus continues to be produced in the middle ear, even though the infection may have cleared up. This can lead to serous otitis and gradual hearing loss which can be remedied with the correct treatment (see below).

Very rarely the eardrum will burst during an ear infection, causing discharge from the ear and a reduction in the intense pain. In most cases the eardrum will heal up completely with a course of antibiotics.

Treatment   Viruses probably cause over half of all ear infections, but in practice it is impossible for doctors to distinguish between a bacterial or viral cause. For this reason all diagnosed ear infections are treated with antibiotics. If your child is prescribed antibiotics it is important to make sure that he takes the full course to prevent recurrence, even if his earache disappears half way through.

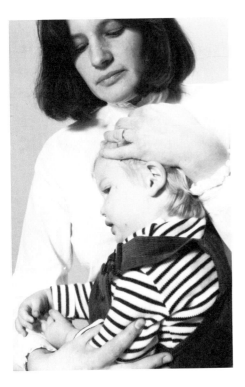

This position will be least stressful for
your child during an ear examination.

To help reduce the pain of the earache straightaway you can give acetaminophen with the antibiotic for the first twenty-four hours, as it will take
that long for the antibiotic to reduce the inflammation and pain. Paracet-
amol given by mouth is much more effective than ear drops. In fact, putting
drops of warm oil into an infected ear is positively dangerous.

If your child has a runny nose as well as earache try taking him out for
a walk. Fresh cool air dries up secretions in the nose and the Eustachian
tubes, which drain the secretions of the middle ear into the back of the
throat. In my experience it is better than medicine!

If your child has fever with the earache, follow the advice on pages
66–70. The infection should clear up with treatment in three to ten days.
Your child should be examined by the doctor once all the symptoms are
gone to make sure the infection is over.

Occasionally, when examining your child for earache, your doctor will
discover that his ears are filled up with excess wax. This does not cause
pain but may affect his hearing and make ear examinations more difficult.
Once your doctor has confirmed that the ear infection has been cleared up
with antibiotics, you can remove the wax with an over-the-counter ear
drop preparation containing glycerine and bicarbonate. First heat up the

bottle in a saucer of warm water, draw up some of the liquid in a dropper, then squeeze a few drops on to the back of your hand to check the temperature; then insert a few drops into the affected ear(s). Your child should hold his head on one side for two minutes to allow the warm liquid to penetrate and dissolve the wax. This procedure needs to be carried out three times a day for at least a week.

To prevent wax building up in the ear, wash your child's ears out with soap once a week in the bath. Do not use sticks tipped with cotton wool to clear wax, as you risk damaging the eardrum.

Serous otitis

This condition may follow repeated ear infections but its cause is not known. Usually the discharge in the Eustachian tube and middle ear drains away after an infection, but in this condition the middle ear gradually fills with sticky mucus, preventing sound waves from moving the drum which normally transmits sound to the nerve endings in the inner ear.

Serous otitis may first be discovered during a hearing test at around the age of two to three years, or it may be found as a result of impaired hearing more than three months after an ear infection. Sometimes the condition is not noticed until school age, although it only occurs extremely rarely after the age of seven or eight.

Symptoms   Unlike the ear infection which preceded it, serous otitis does not cause fever, and is usually not painful. The main symptom is impaired hearing, which varies from total deafness to deafness in one ear or inability to hear high tones like the sound made by the letter 's'. Anything less than total deafness may pass unnoticed for a long time.

Serous otitis usually builds up gradually and your child's hearing may fluctuate. Some weeks it may be normal, others it may be severely impaired. That is why it is sometimes not detected at a routine screening test, giving parents a false sense of security.

Hearing problems caused by this condition can lead to your child becoming slow at learning and he may seem to 'switch off' during lessons. This blankness may sometimes be misinterpreted as a mild form of epilepsy. These problems at school may eventually result in disruptive behaviour in class.

Opposite: A grommet inserted into the eardrum of children with acute serous otitis helps to clear the inner ear of sticky mucus and improves hearing.

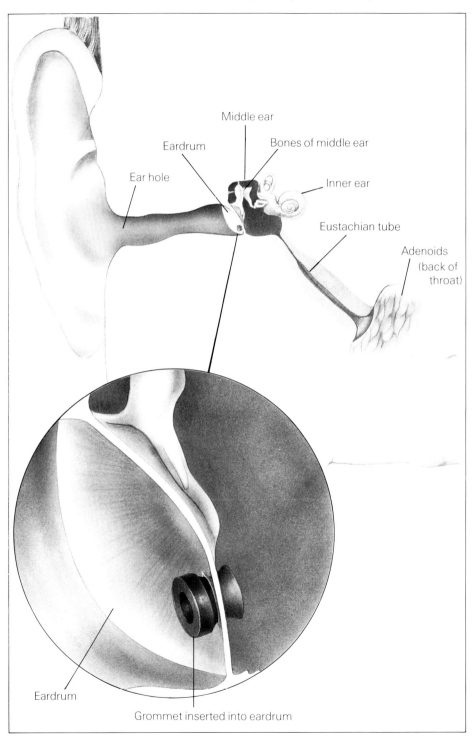

Middle ear

Eardrum

Bones of middle ear

Ear hole

Inner ear

Eustachian tube

Adenoids (back of throat)

Eardrum

Grommet inserted into eardrum

Treatment If serous otitis is suspected your child should be seen by an ear, nose and throat surgeon. After excluding the possibility of deafness due to other causes, he or she will probably wait for a month to six weeks to see if the mucus inside the ear disperses of its own accord. If it does not, a small operation under general anaesthetic is needed, first to suck out the discharge which is causing the deafness and then to insert a tiny plastic drainage tube, called a grommet, into the eardrum. This allows air into the inner ear to dry up any further secretions. Your child will only need to spend one night in the hospital at most. Many of these operations are performed as day cases.

When the grommet is in, your child should avoid putting his head under water.

The grommet usually becomes blocked about six to nine months after insertion. If it does not drop out of its own accord, a second small operation may be needed to remove the grommet, after which the eardrum heals up completely. Rarely serous otitis recurs and another minor operation to reinsert a grommet may be required.

Sometimes the adenoids – small pads of tissue at the back of the nose – block the Eustachian tube, contributing to the development of this condition. If the surgeon finds this to be the case he or she will remove the adenoids (which are dispensable) at the same time as inserting grommets. This may entail your child staying in the hospital for about two days.

Tonsillitis

Inflammation of the tonsils – the two visible pads of tissue that lie on each side of the throat – is very common in children. Tonsillitis is usually due to a virus, and only occasionally to bacteria.

Symptoms In babies fever and refusal of feeds may be the only symptoms, while older children will have a sore throat and swollen red tonsils, possibly covered with white spots. Occasionally there is swelling of the gland under the jaw, which may be confused with mumps (see Chapter 3).

Viral tonsillitis often produces two peaks of fever with one fever-free day in between, which might be misinterpreted as two separate illnesses.

Possible complications The germ causing the tonsillitis may spread back up the Eustachian tubes to infect the ears, causing earache due to otitis media (see previously in this chapter).

Rarely the fever associated with tonsillitis causes a febrile convulsion (see Chapter 3).

Treatment Tonsillitis usually lasts for one to three days, and if your child's temperature does not exceed 102°F (39°C) during this time there is no need for him to see the doctor. You can give acetaminophen or aspirin

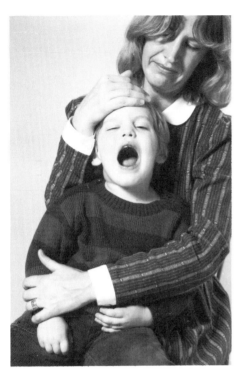

Children dislike having their throats examined even more than their ears.

to ease the pain. Give plenty of fluids to drink, especially milk, which won't irritate your child's sore throat, as fruit juice might. If he wants to eat solid food, give it to him about half an hour after he has taken the painkiller so that swallowing won't be such an ordeal. There is no need to keep your child in bed or even indoors. Treat the fever as described on pages 66–70.

If the fever rises above 102°F (39°C), or if the infection lasts longer than three days, or your infant refuses to drink, he should be seen by the doctor. Children and infants dislike having their throats examined even more than their ears. The easiest way for the doctor to look down your child's throat is if you sit him on your knee and hold his forehead firmly, with the back of his head against your chest (see photograph above).

If your doctor suspects or confirms a bacterial infection, he or she will prescribe penicillin or some other antibiotic for ten days. As with all antibiotics it is very important to complete the course to avoid recurrence of the infection.

Having the tonsils out   If your child has three bouts of bacterial tonsillitis in one year, his ear, nose and throat specialist may decide that it is best to remove the tonsils with a minor surgical operation called a tonsillectomy.

But this operation is rarely performed today, as research has shown that most children outgrow their symptoms by the following winter. A tonsillectomy will not, as many people believe, always cure a recurrent sore throat.

A tonsillectomy would certainly be carried out in the rare event that your child's tonsils became so enlarged that they met in the middle between attacks of infection, blocking the throat.

Croup

This is the popular name for acute laryngitis, which is a viral inflammation of the larynx, or voice box, in the middle respiratory tract. It can be a dangerous infection because it causes narrowing and sometimes obstruction of the airway. Croup most commonly affects infants between six months and two years of age. It is rare in children over five.

Symptoms   Sometimes preceded by cold-like symptoms of feeling unwell and having a runny nose, the distinctive features of croup are noisy breathing, cough and a hoarse voice. The main symptoms often come on suddenly at night and are most severe in the early hours of the morning.

Difficulty with breathing shown by indrawing of the spaces between the ribs, blueness of the lips or drowsiness are signs of severe illness. As there is the risk that the narrowest part of the child's airway can be closed completely by the infection you should phone your doctor immediately if you suspect croup, even if it's the middle of the night. If you can't get hold of him or her and the symptoms are severe, call an ambulance or drive straight to your nearest hospital's emergency room.

Treatment   While waiting for the doctor, take your infant to the bathroom, turn on the hot water tap and get your child to inhale the steam. This will improve the symptoms quickly. Your doctor will decide whether your infant needs to be admitted to the hospital in order to receive increased humidity in a special plastic tent. If your child stays at home you must carefully monitor his condition at all times of the day and night, and make sure he gets to the hospital quickly if it becomes worse. This is definitely an occasion to call on other members of the family for support.

If your child goes to the hospital and his condition deteriorates to the point where his breathing is threatened by the narrowing of the airway, the doctor will insert a plastic tube down the throat and into the airway to bypass the obstruction and ensure trouble-free breathing. The tube will need to be kept in place for between one and seven days.

Antibiotics are useless against this infection, as it is caused by a virus. The only thing to be done is to wait for the infection to pass – sometimes this takes twenty-four hours, sometimes several days – and make sure your child is under observation until out of danger. Though distressing at the time, croup has no lasting ill effects.

Epiglottitis
The epiglottis is a flap of skin below the back of the tongue, which can become infected with bacteria. If it becomes severely inflamed it may swell, partially obstructing the main airway and threatening to close it off completely. This life-threatening condition produces symptoms similar to those of severe croup (opposite) and in all cases urgent medical help is needed. Call an ambulance if necessary.

Epiglottitis is always treated in the hospital. Antibiotics usually clear up the inflammation within a few days, but your child will be kept under careful observation, especially during the first twenty-four hours, before the antibiotic has had time to take effect. As with croup, a plastic tube may need to be inserted down the windpipe if the airway becomes obstructed.

Similar symptoms to croup and epiglottitis can be produced by a foreign body such as a peanut or small object lodged in your infant's airway. If he has persistent noisy breathing after choking over food or playing around with a small object, telephone your doctor immediately for emergency advice and treatment.

Coughing
The main symptom of infections affecting the lower respiratory tract is recurrent coughing. Bronchitis is a common minor ailment of childhood, whereas bronchiolitis and pneumonia are rarer and more serious illnesses that need to be treated in the hospital.

Acute bronchitis   This condition most commonly affects children in the one- to four-year-old age group, when the breathing tubes in the lung are small. If your child has wheezing with a cough, the larger tubes of his lung may be inflamed. With acute bronchitis there is usually no fever, nor difficulty with feeding. The symptoms usually disappear within a week without treatment or special care, and do not need the attention of your doctor, unless your baby is under one year of age. In this case his condition should be watched closely in case it becomes worse, as it may be due to bronchiolitis, which can be dangerous (see overleaf).

Your child can continue with all his usual activities. Plenty of fresh air will probably hasten complete recovery by helping to dry up the mucus secreted by the lungs, and is much more effective than any over-the-counter inhalants or chest rubs.

Recurrent bronchitis   In some children viral infections appear to go straight down into the chest rather than be confined to the nose. These infants have an episode of cough with or without wheezing whenever they have a cold. They usually do not feel ill during these episodes, no special care is needed, and antibiotics are rarely prescribed. Recurrent bronchitis is most common during the second half of a child's first year of life, his first two years at kindergarten or nursery school, or his first two years at primary school. But the chance of developing these attacks for the first time will lessen as your child approaches the age of four years.

If your child has three or more attacks during one year, as commonly happens, it may be advisable for you to go back to your doctor for further investigations in order to exclude the possibility of an underlying condition such as cystic fibrosis or asthma (see opposite). Most infants with recurrent bronchitis will lose all their symptoms by the age of four but in a few the symptoms may persist, suggesting at that age the presence of asthma (see later in this chapter).

Acute bronchiolitis   This condition is the most serious viral respiratory infection and the most common cause of abrupt deterioration in an infant who was previously well. It is an infection of the lungs which occurs in winter epidemics in infants aged under a year, and most commonly in the under-six-months age group.

Following a cough which may be mild for the first few days, the distinctive signs of bronchiolitis are drowsiness and refusal to feed. The infant with bronchiolitis always breathes faster than normal and may have fever.

Infants with these symptoms should be seen by a doctor that day, especially if they are under six months of age. Some will be admitted to the hospital and carefully monitored for a few days, as it may not be possible for your doctor to determine whether your child's bronchiolitis will get worse after a first examination.

If your infant's condition does deteriorate, he will be placed in a plastic oxygen tent to help his breathing and will be fed either via a tube inserted painlessly down the nose and into the stomach, or via a drip into a vein. Antibiotics will not help, as bronchiolitis is always caused by a virus, but his condition will be watched closely for five to ten days – the time the infection takes to run its course. Nearly all infants who have severe bronchiolitis recover completely, although the cough may persist for up to a month until the lungs are completely better. Fortunately you can only catch this disease once.

Pneumonia is an uncommon acute inflammation of the lung which may be caused by either viruses or bacteria, and may follow a cold. Pneumonia is not caused, as many people still believe, by being out in the cold with wet hair or damp clothes. Whereas bronchiolitis (see above) tends to affect infants under six months old, pneumonia nearly always affects children over that age.

The high rate of breathing at rest distinguishes it from ordinary bronchitis. There is also cough, difficulty in feeding and sometimes fever. If your child has these symptoms he should be seen by a doctor as soon as possible.

Children with pneumonia are best treated in the hospital as they often need oxygen to help with breathing, as well as other forms of treatment, such as a course of antibiotics, which will be started straight away, as a precautionary measure in case the infection is bacterial. Physiotherapy might also be given to help bring mucus up from the lungs (see page 62). As during hospital treatment for acute bronchiolitis (opposite) your child may be fed via a tube going from the mouth to the stomach or via a drip into an arm vein. In nearly all cases of pneumonia recovery is complete. Your child will be feeling better in five to ten days, but it may take three or four weeks before his cough disappears and his lungs recover fully.

Asthma

This condition affects 5–10 per cent of children. It causes attacks of coughing, wheezing and tightness of the chest, especially after exercise and during the night. Asthma tends to run in families and some asthmatic children may also suffer from either eczema (see Chapter 6) or hay fever (see overleaf) or both. If you suspect asthma, take your child to the doctor. If three episodes have occurred within a year, the diagnosis of asthma is likely. The first attack can occur at any age but it may be difficult for doctors as well as parents to distinguish between asthma and recurrent bronchitis (see page 91), especially if your child is below the age of three.

The symptoms of asthma are caused by narrowing of the breathing tubes due to swelling of their lining; mucus obstructing the middle of the tube; and contraction of the muscles surrounding the tube. Most asthmatic children have no symptoms between attacks.

Trigger factors

Infection Most asthma attacks in children are believed to be triggered off by viral infection such as colds, so antibiotics are not helpful.

Exercise is a common trigger factor in children, especially if taken in cold dry air. Your doctor may ask your child to exercise when examining him to see if this brings on wheezing.

Swimming in a heated indoor pool is a particularly good form of exercise for asthmatics, as the warm humid environment is less likely to start an attack.

Psychological stress The exact role of stress in starting attacks of asthma is not clear. It is a 'chicken-and-egg' problem. It is true that many children are under psychological stress when they have an acute asthma attack, but it is difficult to know whether it was the stress which caused the attack, whether their asthmatic condition was the cause of the stress, or, as is most

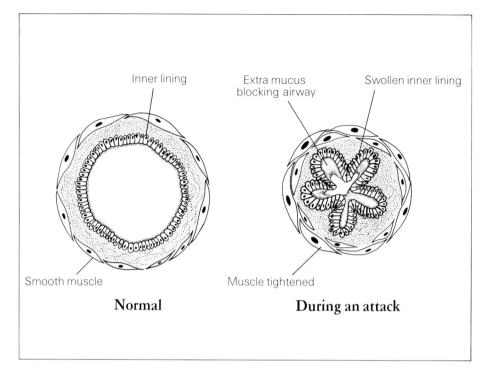

A cross-section of a bronchial tube, showing what happens during an asthmatic attack.

likely, it was a combination of the two – a vicious circle. Modern drug treatments for asthma are probably the best way to break this circle and I describe these below.

Allergy   Your child's asthma may be an allergic reaction to one or more of several common substances in the environment. For example, if your child has an attack whenever he goes to stay with his grandmother who has a dog, he may be found to have an allergy to dog fur. Pet cats, rodents, birds, and horses are also capable of causing problems for asthmatic children.

The microscopic house dust mite which inhabits bed clothes, soft furnishings and cuddly toys is one of the commonest culprits for setting off asthma attacks.

If severe asthma symptoms or hay fever with a runny nose and watering eyes occur at a particular time each year, pollens from grasses or trees, or mold spores may be responsible.

Skin prick tests
These may be given by your doctor to try to find out to which, if any, of

these factors your child is allergic. This is a painless procedure in which very diluted extracts of several of the commonest allergy trigger substances, or allergens, are inserted into your child's skin on the point of a fine needle. If he is allergic to any of the substances a small reddened area will usually appear around the pin prick within fifteen minutes. The skin-prick test is not so useful in children under five years of age as their skin may show no reaction even though they may be allergic to one or more of the substances they have been tested with.

Desensitization
Desensitization involves giving shots containing minute doses of the allergen to stimulate your child's immune system into producing high levels of antibodies to combat the allergen. The long-term effectiveness of this technique, which is similar in principle to immunization (see Chapter 3), is not known, but we do know that it is not as successful as currently available drug therapy (see below).

Avoiding allergens
House dust, house dust mite and grass pollens produce the highest number of positive skin prick tests in children with asthma. Complete avoidance of house dust and house dust mite is obviously impossible but you can help to reduce house dust mite levels by replacing your child's feather pillows with foam rubber pillows, his feather-filled duvet with one containing a synthetic filling and by completely enclosing his mattress in a plastic bag. It may be helpful to use damp dusters for wiping surfaces and to clean your child's room only while he is in another part of the house. Don't forget that old furry cuddly toys also make an ideal home for the house dust mite.

Drug treatment
Today's drugs against asthma, introduced over the last decade or so, are safe and effective and should enable your child to lead a completely normal life. If properly controlled, his asthma should not prevent him from joining in sports and physical exercises at school. Should he start wheezing during exercise or be woken by coughing and wheezing in the middle of the night despite taking his medicine as advised, take him back to the doctor to have his treatment reviewed rather than stop him from doing what he enjoys.

Drugs prescribed for asthma are divided into those which reduce the symptoms during attacks and those used continuously to prevent attacks from starting in the first place.

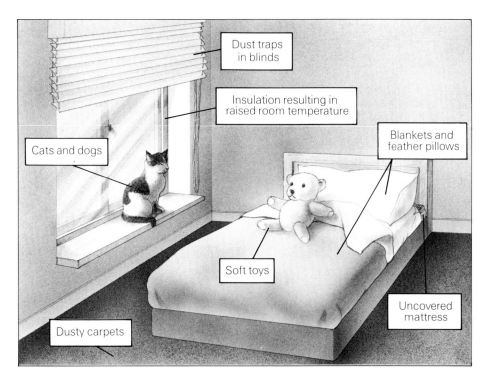

Watch out for these danger spots in your child's bedroom. These places are likely to harbour house dust and mites which may provoke attacks.

For treating attacks   During mild attacks a bronchodilator drug, such as salbutamol, which widens, or dilates, the bronchial tubes in the lung, can be given as a syrup, pill or inhaled powder. The same type of medicine can be given half an hour before strenuous exercise to prevent symptoms from occurring.

Your doctor may advise you to monitor your child's asthma by using a peak flow meter to measure how deeply your child can breathe out (see opposite). Because peak flow often declines gradually before an attack, this technique can give prior warning of trouble and enable you to abort the attack before it starts by giving a prescribed dose of bronchodilator drug, as advised by your doctor.

For long-term prevention   If your child is breathless after mild exercise or has recurrent episodes of asthma more frequently than once every two months he may need a preventive drug continuously for at least a year. Cromolyn Sodium has been used for over twelve years and is effective at preventing asthma in most children with the condition if taken two or

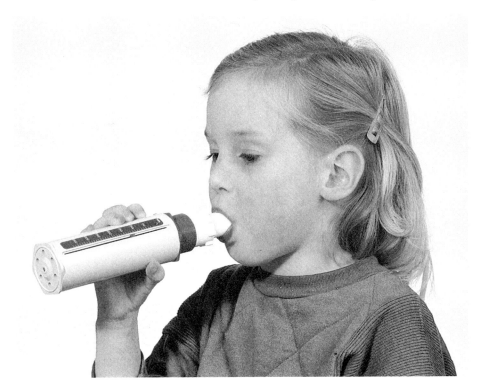

This portable mini peak flow meter will give prior warning of an asthmatic attack, if used regularly.

three times a day. It is not suitable for treating actual attacks, when a bronchodilator such as salbutamol should be used. Rarely, the powder irratates the throat and causes coughing but there are no other side-effects in the short or long term.

Children usually have to be over the age of about four years before they can master the technique of sucking air and powdered cromolyn through the special inhaler and into their lungs. Problems with inhalation technique are a common cause of failure to respond to the drug. If your child continues to have difficulty with the method, ask your doctor or nurse to repeat the instructions. In younger children and those who cannot manage the technique, cromolyn has recently become available as a preparation which can be given as an aerosol via a mask and nebulizer. Taking cromolyn by nebulizer takes about fifteen minutes on each occasion.

An alternative to cromolyn for preventive treatment (particularly in younger children) is one of the long-acting preparations of theophylline, another type of bronchodilator drug. But there is no liquid preparation,

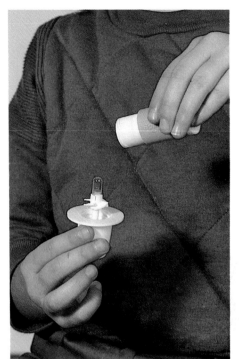 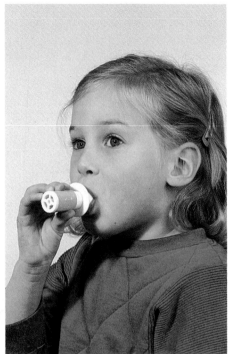

Spinhaler technique: Insert the capsule into the Spinhaler and twist the inhaler collar to pierce the capsule (left). Inhale the powder deeply. Hold your breath for a moment. Repeat if necessary to empty the capsule completely (right).

so either the pills must be swallowed whole, or there is a preparation of theophylline granules which can be taken out of the capsule and spread on jam or other food. Once your child has started theophylline therapy, your doctor will probably take a painless blood test to check the concentration of theophylline in the blood. He can then tailor the dose precisely, to avoid the possible side-effects of vomiting and headaches.

If your child has severe asthma which does not respond to cromolyn or theophylline your doctor will prescribe a steroid powder for inhalation three times daily. Steroids are the most powerful treatment available and are therefore reserved for those children who don't respond to other types of therapy. The dose of steroid is extremely small but works because it reaches the lungs directly and does not have to be absorbed through the bloodstream. This treatment has been used successfully for about eight years. Rarely thrush (candadiasis) occurs in the mouth (see page 17) but there no other side-effects in the short term.

What to do in a severe attack
Drowsiness, blueness of the lips and shortness of breath during speaking

are signs of a severe attack. If your child has these symptoms he must be admitted to the hospital urgently. When he reaches the hospital he will usually receive a bronchodilator such as salbutamol given by aerosol using a face mask and nebulizer attached to an air pump. Even the smallest child can take this treatment well, especially if you, the parent, hold the mask and talk to your child during the treatment.

If the attack is not stopped by a nebulized bronchodilator, your child may be given a shot of theophylline with or without a steroid. Once the attack is over he will probably be allowed to go home. Severe attacks can recur, but the chances are lessened if your child has good preventive treatment as described above. The thing to remember when your child's asthma is depressing or worrying you, is that most youngsters grow out of it by their teens. If you want to know more about asthma, I recommend reading *Asthma and Hay Fever* by Dr Allan Knight, also in this series.

Hayfever

Otherwise known as allergic rhinitis (rhinitis meaning inflammation of the nose), this condition affects about 10 per cent of the population under the age of 20. Common hayfever-provoking allergens include house dust,

A young child under emergency nebulization of bronchodilator in hospital.

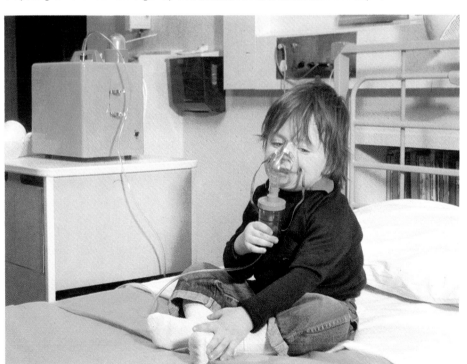

animal fur, pollens, certain foods and food additives. Hayfever can be classified into two types; the commonest – *seasonal rhinitis* – occurs at specific times of the year and can often be pinpointed to one particular allergen, such as grass pollen in Summer; *perennial rhinitis* occurs continuously throughout the year and is provoked by one or more allergens; In the latter case it is often difficult to isolate one allergen as the cause because the symptoms are constant.

Symptoms   The distinctive features of hayfever are similar to a common cold – sneezing; congested nose; itchy, runny nose; red, sore eyes; coughing, especially at night; 'blocked' or 'popping' ears and occasionally glue ear (see page 86).

Prevention and treatment   Advice on avoiding allergens is given on page 95. Your doctor may try to pinpoint specific allergens by performing skin-prick tests or may consider desensitization therapy (see page 95). Or he may place your child on a special diet if a food or food additive is the cause of his hayfever. If drug preparations are necessary, your doctor may prescribe antihistamines, vasoconstrictor drugs, oral decongestants or cromolyn sodium in aerosol form (see page 95). The latter is particularly effective in severe hayfever and is also available as eye drops to help relieve itchy, swollen eyes. Oral decongestants and vasoconstrictors will help to clear a blocked nose and throat.

While on antihistamines or decongestants, your child might feel drowsy or may be irritable or have difficulty sleeping. If you feel your child's performance at school is being affected by the drugs, consult your doctor or pediatrician. Most of the newer preparations however do not have these minor side effects.

Giving medicines

Medicines taken at home for any illness are usually given three times during your child's waking hours. This means that you never have to wake him up especially for his medicines. It's important, of course, to carefully check the dosage regime on the bottle. Some medicines have an unpleasant taste and should not be mixed with food as it might put your child off eating.

If only one parent is available to give medicine to the baby, wrapping him securely in a blanket may prevent spillage.

If your child is particularly difficult or if you have to give very small amounts of medicine, you can measure the medicine in a special syringe (without a needle) and squirt it into your child's mouth.

All medicines should be locked in a cupboard with a key that is inaccessible to toddlers, as most drugs are potentially dangerous if taken in excessive amounts.

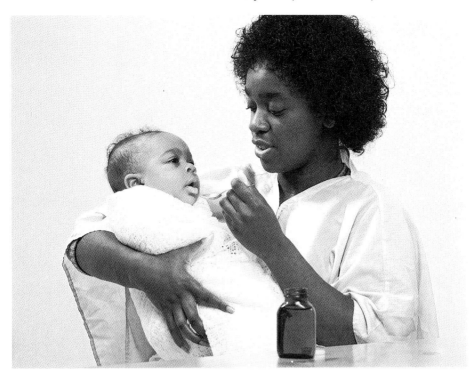

You will find it easier to give a young baby medicine by wrapping him securely in a blanket.

Eye problems

As I mentioned in Chapter 1, a normal newborn baby can focus on his mother's face when breast-feeding or held at arm's length, even during the first week of life. At that age he tends to move his eyes in short, jerky movements, which are normal. Minor eye ailments that are common in babies include watering eyes (see page 21) and conjunctivitis, which is an inflammation of the conjunctiva, or transparent membrane covering the eyelids and whites of the eye. Conjunctivitis affects older children too. The main symptoms are redness of the eye with sticky discharge and treatment is the same as described on page 20.

Lazy eye
It is believed that around 5 to 8 per cent of children have a strabismus (also called a squint) – the commonest children's eye problem. You should suspect this condition if one eye seems to be looking at an object while the other always looks in another direction. Sometimes a baby's eyes will

move in an uncoordinated way, but this is only due to normal immaturity of eye movement. If your child has a strabismus you can see that light will fall in a different place on each pupil, the black spot in the center of the eye.

A strabismus present from birth will probably be noticed at the routine tests of vision given at your infant's first checkup after leaving the hospital. The doctor will observe whether your baby moves his eyes normally in response to a moving object or the examiner's face. Most often, though, a strabismus first becomes apparent later in life – when your child is tired – either between the ages of two and three when he starts to focus on close objects or when he goes to school.

If you suspect a strabismus at any age take your child to the doctor. Early diagnosis and treatment are particularly important with this condition. Often the eye that is out of alignment causes double vision. To cut out the conflicting images, that eye gradually 'switches off', and becomes 'lazy'. In some types of strabismus, by the age of seven or eight years the eye totally loses its ability to see.

The doctor will check the movements of the eyes by covering each eye separately. If he thinks further tests are necessary before a diagnosis is made he may advise you to take your child to a eye doctor – an ophthalmologist – or to an optometrist – a specialist who has a particular interest in the diagnosis and treatment of strabismi.

Some infants have what is called a false squint due to the wide space between their eyes, or to the folds of skin on the inner edge of their eyelids. A false squint is most noticeable in early infancy, and gradually disappears as your child's face grows.

Treatment   Once a true strabismus is confirmed, your child will need specialist treatment. Children do not, as is widely believed, grow out of a true strabismus. Your child will need to be seen by an ophthalmologist.

Treatment may involve covering one eye temporarily with a patch to make the 'lazy' eye work harder. Two-thirds of strabismi need a small operation to alter the length of one of the muscles attached to the eye. The age at which these operations are performed depends on the severity of the strabismus and the personal practice of the surgeon. Your child might be allowed home on the same day of the operation, or he might have to stay in the hospital for a night or two. He will need to have a pad over his eye for a few days, and his eye will be red and a little sore for about a month. But he will not be in bad pain.

In some children a squint is caused by defective vision in one or both eyes. If this is the case with your child, the defect may be able to be corrected with glasses, which should be worn as much of the time as possible. Most children will tolerate wearing glasses from the age of eighteen months, or even earlier. But if yours won't, contact lenses can be used, even for babies.

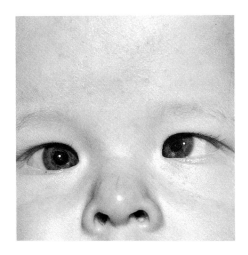

A convergent strabismus with the left eye turned inwards.

1.

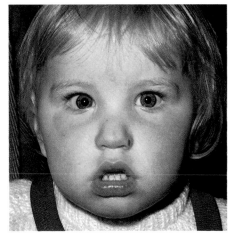

2.

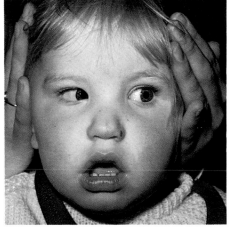

A false or 'pseudo' strabismus:
1. When the child looks straight ahead, the eyes are normal.

2. When the child looks to the side, it gives the impression of a strabismus, but it is due to the child's wide nose and not to an eye defect.

Defective vision

Some children are born with defective vision. They may be far-sighted, not being able to focus on objects close to them; or near-sighted, not being able to focus on objects in the distance; or they may have other problems.

Defective vision might not be noticed for several years because your child may think that everyone sees as he sees, and that it is normal not to be able to focus clearly. The first signs that your child cannot see properly may be noticed at around the age of three or four when he shows no interest in books or watching television. His disability could lead to lack of interest or even disruptive behavior at school, due to not being able to read either his school books, or the blackboard.

Routine tests of visual acuity, that is, how good your child's vision is, are usually performed just before or just after starting school. Your child will be asked to read aloud letters of decreasing size from a card. This test may not show up every type of visual defect, so if at any time you suspect your child is not seeing as well as he should, consult your doctor, optician or optometrist.

5. ABDOMINAL, URINARY AND GENITAL PROBLEMS

Diarrhea

Diarrhea is the passage of loose stools more often than you would expect from the diet and age of your baby or child. It is a definite change in bowel habit. When diarrhea is severe the stools may be mistaken for urine.

As we saw in Chapter 1, the normal stools of a breast-fed baby are never solid, may be passed at hourly intervals, may contain mucus and may be green. And when the milk supply becomes established between the third and fifth days, frequent stools are common and are not due to illness.

Gastroenteritis

The most common cause of acute diarrhea in babies and children is gastro-enteritis which is due to an infection affecting the small intestine. Most infants have at least one attack of gastroenteritis, but it is less common in babies who are breast-feeding. The commonest germ causing gastroenteritis in children is a particular virus called the rotavirus. Scandinavian research in 1977 showed that the virus is probably spread by adults (usually members of the family) who carry the germ without having any symptoms of the disease. Sometimes gastroenteritis is caused by poor sterilization of bottle-feeding equipment, but now sterilization techniques are so good this is not as common as the breath-borne rotavirus infection. If your baby comes down with gastroenteritis, you shouldn't feel guilty about not sterilizing properly, as this is probably not the cause.

Symptoms   The illness has an incubation period of twenty-four to forty-eight hours. It often begins with stomach pains and/or fever with or without ear infection or cough (see Chapter 4), and the diarrhea and vomiting start a few days later. The vomiting lasts from one to three days and usually the stools return to normal after around five days.

The main danger of gastroenteritis is dehydration and loss of various salts which are essential to body function. In addition your child will be very infectious to other infants in the family, ward or nursery. Gastroenter-itis is particularly dangerous to infants under the age of six months.

When to see the doctor   Any infant under the age of six months who has gastroenteritis should be seen by a doctor, whereas older children with a mild attack need not be. As long as there are no worrying symptoms of severe illness you can keep your child at home and follow the advice on treatment given below.

Serious symptoms in children of any age which need a doctor's attention without delay are:

- Vomiting of all fluids given
- Unusual drowsiness
- Loss of 5 per cent of body weight
- Sunken eyes
- Inelastic skin
- Dry tongue
- Not passing urine for several hours
- Persistent diarrhea despite following the recommendations below.

These are signs that your child needs urgent admission to the hospital.

Treatment Antibiotics do not help in gastroenteritis, so the virus has to be eliminated by the body. The main principle of treatment for children of any age is to keep your child well hydrated until he recovers spontaneously. If he is being cared for in the hospital, he may be given fluid via a drip directly into a vein in the arm. If you are looking after him at home stop all milk and solids for twenty-four hours and give him only rehydrating fluid.

The ideal rehydrating fluid is a mixture containing a sugar and various salts that are lost in the diarrhea. Use 2½ level teaspoonfuls (12 g) of granulated sugar in 6 fl oz (200 ml) of water. It is vital to remember that it is dangerous to add salt to the mixture.

Infants under the age of six months need 2½ fl oz of rehydrating fluid for each pound of body weight (150 ml for every kilogram) in twenty-four hours. Older children should be given as much to drink as they wish and will usually need between 2 and 2½ pt (1 and 1.5 l) in twenty-four hours. Vomiting may be reduced by giving small volumes of rehydrating fluid every half an hour.

After twenty-four hours you can reintroduce milk diluted to a quarter of its normal strength for infants under six months, gradually increasing to full strength within four days. When your baby's vomiting has stopped and he is showing signs of hunger you can start him on fruit or vegetable purées if he was previously eating solids. He can return completely to his usual diet once he is receiving full-strength milk.

For infants and children over six months of age food can gradually be reintroduced after twenty-four hours on the rehydrating fluid if vomiting has stopped and some degree of appetite has returned. But milk and milk products such as cheese and yogurt should be excluded from the diet for one week and then be reintroduced gradually.

The main cause of persistent symptoms and subsequent admission to the hospital is failure to follow the above plan of treatment, but a small proportion of infants have temporary damage to the surface of the gut which makes them intolerant to cows' milk preparations for several weeks or even months. These infants may need a special diet which excludes cows' milk preparations (see below).

Chronic diarrhea
Diarrhea which lasts longer than two weeks can be called chronic. It should always be investigated by a doctor.

'Toddlers' diarrhea'   In developed countries chronic diarrhea in children with normal growth (see chart on page 34) between the ages of one and three years usually has no sinister significance. Popularly known as 'toddlers' diarrhea', it is probably due to failure to chew food. You will be able to see recognizable foods such as beans, peas, corn, carrots or raisins in the stool. 'Toddlers' diarrhea' is harmless and you do not need to take any preventive measures. Your child will grow out of it in time.

Cows' milk protein intolerance   Gastroenteritis (see above) may be followed by chronic diarrhea; intolerance to the protein in cows' milk is thought by experts to be the most probable cause. This type of diarrhea starts between the ages of birth and six months and affects only around 1 child in 1,000.

A normal rate of weight gain (see chart on page 34) excludes the poss- ibility that your infant has an underlying ailment such as celiac disease that prevents his small intestine from absorbing food (see below). Your doctor's diagnosis of cows' milk protein intolerance depends on his withdrawing all products containing cows' milk from your infant's diet for a few days and then giving him 1 teaspoon (5 ml) of milk under close supervision. Simple as it sounds, this is a medical procedure which should not be tried as a self-help measure. If diarrhea recurs within forty-eight hours the diagnosis is confirmed and he will prescribe a cows'-milk-free diet to be supervised by a dietitian. Your child's dietitian will make sure that he gets sufficient protein from other sources to sustain his growth. Babies under the age of one year may need a milk substitute and a soy-based preparation is often used, although up to half these children eventually become intol- erant of it and get diarrhea again.

A small volume of cows' milk will be given to your child every two to three months until he can tolerate it without the diarrhea returning. Usually this happens by the age of two years.

Tests for an underlying illness   If your child has chronic diarrhea, is under one year old and is not gaining weight as fast as he should, your doctor will recommend that certain specialist tests be performed to rule out the possibility of an underlying disease.

His stools will be examined for bacteria, blood will be taken for a blood count and a sweat test will be performed, because in cystic fibrosis (see below) sweat has a high salt content. In this test a piece of paper is placed on your child's forearm, covered with plastic and he is allowed to sweat into the paper. The paper is then taken off and the amount of salt estimated in the laboratory. He may be given other tests as well. If none of them bring to light any problems your child will be admitted to hospital for what is called a jejunal biopsy to find out whether he has celiac disease (see below). In this test, which is carried out under sedation, a minute scraping of the surface of the small intestine is obtained by passing a special capsule attached to a thin suction tube through the mouth into the intestine. The procedure is carried out while your child is sedated. It takes from a few minutes to a couple of hours and does not hurt. Your child may be allowed home on the same day, or may need to stay in the hospital for up to two nights.

Cystic fibrosis   This is a life-long inherited ailment that affects around 1 child in 2,000. At present there is no method for diagnosing the condition in the fetus during pregnancy and no reliable screening test in the newborn. In addition to chronic diarrhea, a high sweat salt content, which will be discovered in hospital tests, is a distinctive feature of this condition. If an infant with cystic fibrosis has diarrhea it is due to an abnormality of the pancreas.

The main complication of the disease is recurrent chest infections but if you give your child vigorous physiotherapy at an early age, as advised by a hospital physiotherapist, this may prevent them developing (see page 62). When lung infections occur your doctor will treat them with antibiotics (see page 93). The diarrhea and the problem with the pancreas can be improved under the supervision of a dietitian, who will give advice on a low-fat diet with supplements of pancreatic extract as powder.

Celiac disease (Celiac sprue or gluten sensitive enteropathy)   The jejunal biopsy test described above may reveal that your child's diarrhea is caused by celiac disease, a rare condition affecting around 1 child in 2,000.

In children with celiac disease the surface of the small intestine is flat rather than being composed of multiple finger-like projections. This defect prevents the intestine from absorbing nutrients from food properly, resulting in poor weight gain in infants, accompanied by chronic diarrhea.

Celiac disease is caused by sensitivity to gluten, a protein which is present in wheat and certain other grains, such as rye and barley and possibly oats. When your infant is put on a diet free of gluten under the supervision of a dietitian his symptoms will resolve and he will grow normally. For more information on this subject, see *The Gluten-Free Diet Book*, a companion volume in this series.

Constipation

I mentioned constipation in Chapter 1 as a problem in bottle-fed babies. It affects older children too. Some children's bowel habit is to pass firm stools every two or three days, and this is normal. Constipation only becomes a problem when the stools become hard and difficult to pass and your child's bowel movements become less frequent.

Constipation may be caused by an inadequate intake of fluid or not eating enough solids to form stools during a feverish illness (for recommended fluid intake see page 70); or, more commonly, to a diet lacking in roughage or fiber. To prevent constipation caused by diet, make sure your child eats plenty of fresh fruit and vegetables, and wholewheat brown bread and breakfast cereals. A high-fiber diet alone may not be sufficient to alleviate constipation; you can try giving an over-the-counter laxative, such as pills containing extract of senna, for two or three days.

Anal fissure

Once your child is badly constipated there is the risk of anal fissure, which is a crack in the skin just inside the anus. It is usually due to damage caused by passing a hard stool. The fissure causes severe pain because the area is stretched as each hard stool is being passed. Sometimes this may produce bleeding and you will be able to see fresh red blood on the surface of the stools.

As a result of the pain your child will resist passing stools and so in the end they become harder and the symptoms more severe. Without treatment this vicious circle can lead to long-term constipation (see overleaf).

Treatment If your child has an anal fissure he should see the doctor. Treatment consists of keeping the stools soft, both by ensuring an adequate fluid intake and by giving 5 ml of methylcellulose liquid three times daily for a month and daily for a further month. This preparation can be bought over the counter in pharmacies.

Your child will then be able to regain confidence that passing stools will not be painful. It is essential that this course of treatment is completed, as the fissure takes up to eight weeks to heal.

Surgical removal of the fissure or stretching of the anus is rarely needed if the above treatment is given.

Chronic constipation

While he has an anal fissure your child may hold back his stools by crossing his legs, for example, to avoid the discomfort of passing them. When he eventually passes these stools they may be enormous and cause severe pain. Eventually the whole of the large intestine can become distended with firm stool and the reflex urge to pass stools will be lost as a result of persistent swelling of the rectum. At this stage large masses of feces can be felt through the abdominal wall.

Liquid stool may trickle continuously around the masses and escape with gas through the anus. You might mistake the continual loss of fluid stool for diarrhea if you are unaware of your child's underlying constipation. Fortunately this degree of constipation is not common.

Treatment   Prolonged medical treatment is needed both to empty the bowel and to keep it that way so that it returns to its normal size. Your doctor will probably prescribe a regime containing three different types of laxative, which should be followed regularly for a prolonged period, often up to a year. You can help to encourage the return of the reflex involved in normal passage of stools by asking your child to sit on the lavatory at the same time each day.

This treatment is successful in the vast majority of children with chronic constipation. Suppositories, enemas and the manual removal of feces under anesthetic are rarely necessary.

Acute stomach ache

At the beginning of an attack of stomach ache it may be difficult to be certain whether it is serious or not, especially in children under two years of age. It probably is a cause for concern if your child has accompanying diarrhea, vomiting, fever, rash or pain in the joints, or if he is in such pain that he screams.

Your child should see a doctor if he has stomach ache with any of these symptoms. You don't need to call out your doctor for stomach ache on its own unless it lasts longer than four hours. Most stomach aches which are not serious are gone in four hours. While your child is in pain a hot-water bottle held against the stomach is very soothing, but do not give analgesics as they can mask the pain, making diagnosis more difficult. Also, do not give your child laxatives for stomach aches as they can aggravate an inflamed appendix.

Appendicitis

Inflammation of the appendix, a small, worm-shaped, dead-end tube attached to the large intestine, may produce symptoms common to many other conditions, so your doctor may not find it possible to make a firm diagnosis or to exclude the possibility of appendicitis on one visit. If he thinks appendicitis is likely, he will advise you to withhold solid food, as your child may need an operation.

Appendicitis is extremely rare in infants under three years of age, but around one in every hundred seven-year-olds gets an inflamed appendix.

Medical experts now consider that appendicitis is always acute and that there is no such thing as a 'grumbling' appendix.

Symptoms   Children can often point to the site of their pain with one finger. The pain of appendicitis usually starts around the navel and is followed by vomiting. The pain may be continuous or may stop for half an hour or an hour and recur. It may stop during sleep. After a few hours the pain changes position and moves down into the right lower part of the abdomen. In about a quarter of children with appendicitis the pain is in this position from the beginning. The child with appendicitis usually lies still, as his pain is made worse by movement. If you touch your child's stomach it will be tender.

The pain experienced in appendicitis usually starts around the navel and later moves down around the appendix.

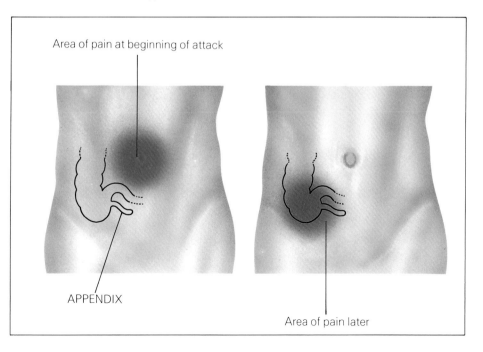

Area of pain at beginning of attack

APPENDIX

Area of pain later

Possible complications   Development of a hole or perforation of the appendix is the most dangerous complication because the bowel contents and their germs are spread around the abdomen, causing severe infection, and continuous pain. Nowadays, fortunately, this complication is rare. Pain is usually present for more than twelve hours before perforation occurs so it is safe to wait for four to six hours after the pain begins before your child is seen by a doctor. If the pain is not due to appendicitis it may get better during this period of time. A perforation of the appendix is treated by immediate surgery followed by a course of antibiotics.

Treatment   In view of the difficulty of diagnosing appendicitis, your child may be admitted to the hospital so that he can be examined repeatedly if the doctors are uncertain about the cause of his pain. In the hospital his urine will be checked for infection, as a urinary tract infection may produce very similar symptoms to those of appendicitis (see page 118). Once the diagnosis of appendicitis is confirmed your child will have a simple operation to remove his appendix, after which he should be allowed home after about a week. No special diet is necessary, although plenty of fluids, fresh fruit and vegetables and wholewheat bread will help him to pass stools without painful straining. He will need to refrain from vigorous athletic activities for about six weeks.

   If he is operated on for a perforation he will need to be fed by a drip into an arm vein, and will be given antibiotics. Recovery may take a little longer than after a straightforward appendix operation.

Intussusception
In this condition part of the bowel telescopes into itself, causing internal bleeding. If the condition is not diagnosed and treated quickly the affected part of the bowel may suffer irreversible damage due to interrupted blood supply and will have to be removed in an operation. Intussusception can occur at any age, although it is most common between the ages of three and eleven months.

Symptoms   A distinctive feature is recurrent attacks of severe screaming, drawing up of the legs and appearing pale. In some episodes your child's pallor is the main symptom. The attack lasts a few minutes and then disappears, to recur about twenty minutes later, although attacks may be more frequent. The symptoms of colic (see Chapter 2) differ from those of intussusception in that colicky babies do not seem repeatedly to get better for a while and then start screaming again. Also, intussusception is more common after three months of age, when colic attacks have usually ceased. One or two loose stools may be passed to begin with, suggesting gastroenteritis (see page 105). Some infants with intussusception vomit greenish-yellow material and may pass blood or blood-stained mucus from the back passage.

If you suspect intussusception, telephone your doctor without delay. Between attacks your infant will appear normal and there may be no symptoms apparent when the doctor examines him.

Treatment   If your doctor diagnoses intussusception he will arrange for your child to be admitted to the hospital immediately. There he may be given a barium enema – a painless injection via a tube into the back passage of a radio-opaque fluid that shows up on X-ray. This not only confirms the doctor's diagnosis, but the pressure of the barium enema may also straighten out the bowel. If it does not, an operation will be needed, after which the problem rarely recurs. Your infant will probably need to stay in the hospital for several days. When he returns home no special diet is needed, nor do you need to restrict his activities in any way. The incision should heal up within ten days.

Recurrent stomach ache

This condition, which is also called the periodic syndrome or abdominal migraine, is diagnosed on the basis of at least three episodes of stomach ache with no physical cause over three months. It is one of the commonest reasons why children are seen by a doctor, and affects at least one child in ten. The symptoms usually begin at the age of five years, though they may appear as early as two years or as late as thirteen. In a 1963 study, of one hundred children investigated in hospital in Bristol, England, only eight were found to have physical causes for the pain, the commonest being kidney problems (see page 118). Anxiety is the commonest cause of recurrent stomach ache and the commonest trigger for attacks of pain is events at school. Recurrent stomach ache is the main way anxiety shows itself in childhood, and although caused by emotional tension and not physical disease the pain is very real and often distressing for the child.

Symptoms   Two-thirds of the children with no physical disease have a central stomach ache around the belly button, whereas pain on one side of the stomach might be due to kidney disease. Even very severe pain causing your child to cry out may be caused by emotional reasons. The pain may occur on a particular day of the week, at weekends or on vacation and these factors may give a clue to the cause of your child's anxiety. About two-thirds of the children have vomiting with the pain and 10 per cent have diarrhea during attacks. A quarter of the children have headaches and 10 per cent have pain in their legs between attacks. In addition, about half the children become pale during attacks and a quarter are sleepy after attacks. Stomach ache with no underlying physical complaint does not usually last longer than six hours continuously, and will not produce symptoms such as blood-stained stools, or blood-stained vomit. If these are present your child may have a serious intestinal problem such as intussusception and needs the prompt attention of a doctor (see opposite).

Seeing the doctor   Your doctor will be as anxious as you are not to miss physical disease in your child. You should make sure that he is seen by the doctor, who will examine him thoroughly and should do so again actually during an attack if the opportunity arises. The doctor may take a specimen of urine to send the laboratory for examination and may decide that other tests are also needed to exclude the possibility of a physical cause. It is important to bear in mind that children with recurrent stomach aches caused by emotional tension may also develop physical disease such as appendicitis (see page 111), and if the pain lasts continuously for more than six hours he should be seen again by a doctor as an emergency.

What can be done?   Once physical disease has been ruled out it is often a relief to the whole family, but you should not forget that your child is experiencing real pain which may be severe, and that he is not pretending.

Medicines are of no help for the vast majority of children with recurrent stomach aches. The key to overcoming the problem lies in discovering the cause of the anxiety and then helping your child to avoid, cope with or come to terms with whatever is bothering him.

His schoolteacher may be able to shed some light on the cause. For example, your child may be being bullied at school, or a chance remark which seemed innocuous to a teacher may have had a devastating effect on your child. Alternatively he may be feeling very hurt by not having been given praise when he thought it was due. Children are very sensitive to injustice, especially from their teachers, whom they tend to revere as godlike. Excessive homework, or going to a large school after a small town school may all produce severe stress. A pressurized child may behave superbly in class and then show his parents the results of his pent-up tension in the form of recurrent stomach aches at home.

Family tensions too can build up your child's emotional stress. Excessive parental pressure to do well at school, for example, or marital discord or separation are all common triggers for recurrent stomach aches.

Once you have identified the source of your child's problem, you should do what you can to alleviate or help him avoid the stress. If he feels his teacher is being unfair, for example, go and see him to discuss and resolve the issue. Your child cannot, of course, be insulated from all stresses, indeed some degree of stress is a necessary stimulant in life, but you should try to remove sources of excessive tension if possible.

If your child has pain every day he may need to be admitted to the hospital for short periods to take the stress off you and your family. The object is to determine whether a change of environment will affect the pain. The pain usually abates in the hospital, though not always, but may become worse again immediately after he returns home.

If none of these approaches is successful, your child, or indeed the whole family, may benefit from psychotherapy carried out by either a psychiatrist or a qualified psychologist. Psychotherapy is nothing more than 'talking treatment' in which your child will be encouraged to talk through his problems by a sympathetic and expert listener. An outsider's insight often helps to resolve seemingly insoluble emotional problems such as recurrent stomach aches.

Some other causes of stomach ache

Hernia in the groin   A swelling in the groin which appears suddenly and comes and goes is likely to be an inguinal hernia. It is most common in infants under one year old. What happens is that part of the intestine slips down the inguinal canal, the path from the abdomen (present in both sexes), down which, in boys, the testicle usually descends to the scrotum before birth. An inguinal hernia may need to be operated on as soon as possible as there is the risk that the affected section of intestine may become strangulated and be deprived of its blood supply.

If your child's hernia is painful or he has a stomach ache this process has probably already begun, and he should be taken to the hospital immediately, where he will probably be operated on straight away. Recovery from the operation will be as described for intussusception on page 112.

Twisted testicle   Every boy who sees a doctor for abdominal pain will have his genitals carefully examined. A tender swollen testicle is a sign that the cord leading from the testicle to the abdomen may be twisted. This can cause severe stomach ache and even vomiting. It mostly affects older boys before puberty but can occur in younger boys and rarely in babies. As with a painful inguinal hernia (above), your child will need to go to the hospital immediately to have an operation to try to prevent permanent damage to the testicle.

Allergic purpura   This is a common condition in children which can occur at any age. Stomach ache may precede, but usually accompanies a purple rash and painful swelling of the knees, ankles, elbows and wrists. The rash, which is not itchy and appears on the arms, legs and buttocks, consists of raised spots containing small leakages of blood, which do not fade if you press them.

Your child should be seen by a doctor, but there are no specific treatments for allergic purpura. You can give your child recommended doses of acetaminophen to alleviate the discomfort in the joints, but he does not need to rest them. The ailment will last three or four days, but he may get a second attack lasting a similar period of time within about a month. After a second attack there will be no recurrence.

Diabetes   Children with undiagnosed diabetes may have stomach ache. They will also have other tell-tale symptoms of diabetes, including excessive thirst and urination. Once the condition has been diagnosed by the doctor your child will be started on insulin therapy which will clear up all the symptoms, including the stomach pain. Diabetes is a life-long condition and you can read more about it in *Diabetes* by Dr Jim Anderson and *The Diabetics' Diet Book* by Dr Jim Mann and the Oxford Dietetic Group, both companion volumes in this series.

Urinary tract infection   See page 118.

Genital and urinary problems

Hydrocele
This is a collection of fluid in the scrotum (the pouch containing the testicles), which gives it a swollen appearance. Hydrocele is often present at birth, and the swelling will increase over the following few weeks. But it can affect older babies and children. Although it is not painful, your infant should be seen as soon as possible by the doctor to confirm the diagnosis. Hydrocele usually resolves spontaneously in a few months, so no treatment is needed.

Undescended testicle
Occasionally the testicles have not descended into the scrotum at birth but are still inside the body where they originated. This is particularly common in babies born early. About 2 per cent of all testicles are undescended at the expected delivery date and spontaneous descent rarely occurs after the age of four months and never after a year.

After the newborn period an active muscle reflex can easily pull the testicles up out of the scrotum making them difficult to feel, especially if your hands are cold. But you will often have noticed whether your baby's testicles are both in the scrotum after a hot bath. If one of your child's testicles has not descended by the age of a year he needs to have a small operation between the ages of two and four years to bring it into the normal position. Your child will probably be allowed home the same day as the operation.

Very rarely it is possible for the cord linking an undescended testicle to the abdomen to be twisted (see page 115). If your child has an undescended testicle, severe stomach ache, vomiting and a swelling in the groin, he should see a doctor immediately in case he needs an operation to save a twisted undescended testicle.

Hypospadias
Rarely a boy is born with the opening for urine on the shaft rather than at the tip of the penis. This is associated with absence of the lower half of the foreskin.

The infant will be seen by a plastic surgeon who will arrange for the appropriate operation to be performed. This will result in a normal-looking and normally functioning penis. It is important that your infant is not circumcised if he has hypospadias, as the upper part of the foreskin is needed for this operation.

Circumcision

In 95 per cent of male babies the foreskin and the tip of the penis are united at birth. It has been found that the foreskin can be retracted by the age of one year in about half the babies and by the age of four years in nine out of ten. But you should not try to retract your baby's foreskin until he is about four years old. Attempts to retract the foreskin earlier are likely to injure the surface, causing bleeding, and circumcision may later become necessary.

Before the age of four years the only medical reasons for circumcision are recurrent infection of the foreskin with pus, and ballooning of the foreskin at the beginning of passing water. Circumcision under general anaesthetic may be performed as a day case, or your infant may need to stay in the hospital for up to two nights. Aftercare varies, so you should ask the surgeon or nursing staff for advice on this.

Many circumcisions are performed as a religious ritual, in Jewish families on the eighth day of life and in Moslem families between the age of three and five years.

Vaginal Discharge

We saw in Chapter 1 that a little discharge in newborn girls is normal and is due to withdrawal of the mother's hormones which were in the fetus's circulation.

Later in life, usually between the age of eighteen months and puberty, a common irritation of the vagina and its opening, called vulvovaginitis by doctors, may cause pain on passing urine, or a yellow stain on the underclothes. Occasionally there may be as thin yellowish-green discharge.

Tests The doctor will probably ask you to collect a fresh specimen of urine in a sterile container after your child has been given a bath. This will be analysed in a laboratory to check whether bacteria are causing a urinary infection. Swabs from the vagina may be taken by the doctor and examined in the laboratory.

Rarely these symptoms are due to threadworms entering the vagina from the anus, so you may be asked to obtain a specimen for examination for threadworm eggs. This is done as follows: when your child wakes in the morning, apply clear adhesive tape several times to the stretched skin around the anus and if any eggs are present, they will stick to it.

In nearly all cases these test are negative, but your doctor may prescribe an antibiotic if an infection is present, or a course of piperazine citrate pills if threadworms are found.

Treatment   In most cases the symptoms of vulvovaginitis will clear up if your child simply has a bath twice a day. But avoid bubble baths, since these, as well as detergents in poorly rinsed underclothes, may cause chemically induced vulvovaginitis.

If the symptoms are persistent and severe despite these measures the cause is usually due to your child having a thin lining to her vagina. Your doctor can prescribe a hormonal estrogen cream to be sparingly applied daily for the first three days and then once a week for a month. This tiny dose thickens the vaginal lining without side-effects and usually clears up and prevents symptoms.

If your child has profuse, offensive, blood-streaked vaginal discharge or symptoms which recur despite taking the above measures, she needs to be examined in hospital under a general anaesthetic to check for a foreign body in the vagina – a bead, for example – which she may have inserted herself and is too embarrassed to mention.

Urinary tract infection

Bacterial infection spreading up the urethra to the bladder, and in some children to the kidneys, may affect about 5 per cent of girls and 3 per cent of boys. Urinary tract infection can occur in children at any age, but early diagnosis and effective treatment are especially important in the under-fives as complications that affect the kidney are most common in this age group.

Symptoms include lethargy, vomiting, slow weight gain, high fever up to 105°F (41°C), pain on passing water, frequency of passing water, stomach ache, or bed-wetting in a child previously dry at night, but sometimes there is only recurrent fever with no other symptoms. An unusual colour of the urine is not a symptom of infection and is probably caused by food coloring. Eating a lot of beetroot, for example, can stain the urine bright pink!

Tests   If your child has one or more of the above symptoms with no obvious cause the doctor will probably have a specimen of urine examined for bacteria. The specimen will be taken before your child takes any antibiotics, as the drugs would get into the urine, making accurate analysis impossible. It is helpful to give your child a bath before collecting the urine specimen in a sterilized container, or bag for babies, as this makes interpretation of the results easier. The specimen will also be tested for glucose, as passing urine frequently may be due to diabetes (see page 115).

All children who have a confirmed urinary tract infection need an ultrasound examination of the kidneys or a special type of X-ray examination of the kidneys called an intravenous pyelogram. In this procedure a radio-opaque dye is injected into a vein. This is no more painful than having a blood sample taken. When the dye reaches the kidneys an X-ray is taken which will show up any abnormality that may be causing the infection.

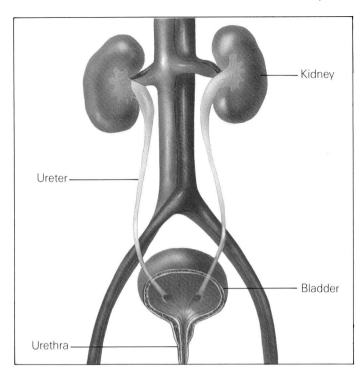

Kidney

Ureter

Bladder

Urethra

The urinary tract.

Treatment usually involves a short course of antibiotics, but in the rare event that infection recurs – sometimes due to a minor abnormality of the kidneys detected by the tests – prolonged low-dose antibiotic treatment may be given. Only very rarely is an operation needed to rectify an abnormality of the kidneys.

6. AILMENTS OF THE SKIN

Rashes usually occur as part of one of the common infectious diseases of childhood (see Chapter 3), and may be confused with some of the skin ailments described in this chapter. A previous attack of an infectious disease makes another attack unlikely, but sometimes a rash due to a skin ailment is wrongly diagnosed as a symptom of an infectious disease, particularly German measles, so that you may be surprised when your child seemingly comes down with the disease twice. The tell-tale clues to the real source of the rash are:

- The characteristics of the spots
- The parts of the body affected
- Changes with time
- Other features of your child's health.

Types of eczema

Childhood eczema
This condition (otherwise known as atopic dermatitis) affects about 1 in 10 of the under-fives, but also occurs in around 1 per cent of schoolchildren. About 70 per cent of children with eczema have a family history of either eczema, asthma or hay fever (see Chapter 4), or a combination of two, or even all three of these conditions, which are known collectively as atopy.

Symptoms Eczema usually appears between the ages of two and six months. You will first notice itching, red, weeping, blistering areas, particularly on the face, in the cracks of the elbows and behind the knees. In severe cases the trunk is also affected. The condition waxes and wanes with or without treatment, and there is often a reduction of symptoms between the ages of two and four years. If the rash has been present for a long time the skin gradually becomes thickened and the outer layer continuously flakes off.

Aggravating factors Some children's eczema is worse during the cold weather and others' skin flares up when it is hot and humid; but moving to a different climate will not necessarily help. Woollen clothing also

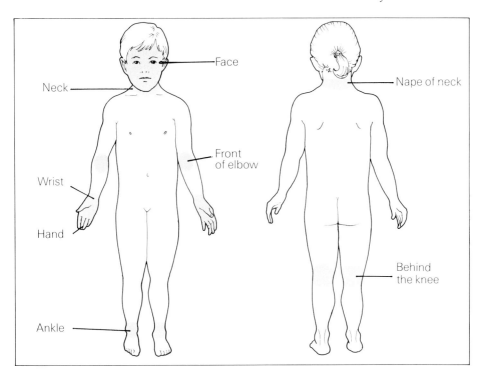

The areas of the body most likely to be affected by childhood eczema.

irritates the skin. Changing your child's diet will not help unless there is clear evidence, confirmed by your doctor, that one or more specific foods make your child's eczema worse. In that case his diet should be supervised by a professional dietitian. An allergy to a specific food is not as common as is widely believed but the usual culprits are high-protein food such as milk, eggs and fish.

Treatment involves thinly applying prescribed anti-inflammatory steroid creams, which should be reduced in strength after about ten days. The aim is to reduce the inflammation, making your child's skin as normal as possible, and to keep it that way using the minimum of treatment.

Different strength steroid creams are prescribed for eczema on different parts of the body, the weakest type being used on the face. It is very important not to mix them up and use a strong steroid meant for the legs on your child's face, for instance.

There are several other ways in which you can help alleviate the discomfort and itch caused by eczema:

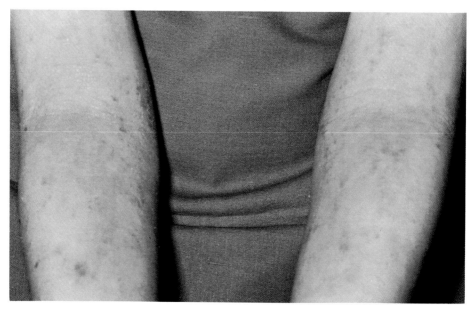

Above: Atopic eczema on the fronts of the elbows.

Left: The areas of the body most likely to be affected by seborrheic dermatitis.

*Above right:*To prevent diaper rash, apply generous amounts of a barrier preparation.

Right: Multiple warts.

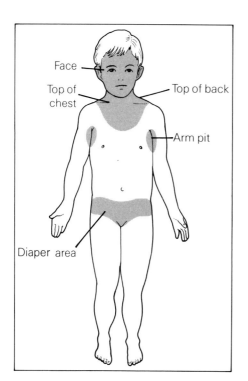

Face

Top of chest

Top of back

Arm pit

Diaper area

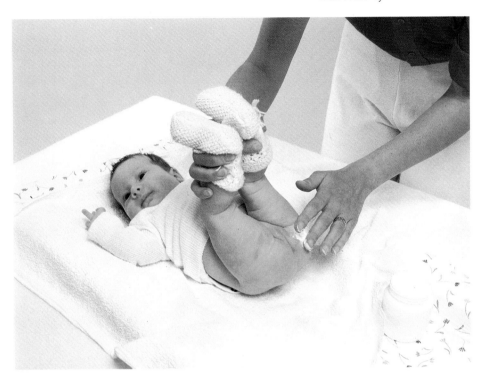

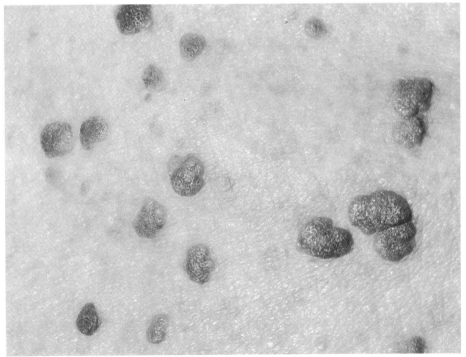

- Frequent baths tend to dry out the skin and make it uncomfortable. Cut down the number of baths and use a prescribed emulsifying ointment or lotion for cleaning the skin, or for moistening it after a bath – aqueous cream, for example.
- Itching may be lessened by adding half a cup of a processed oatmeal to a bath of tepid water.
- Itching at night can be diminished by giving a prescribed antihistamine medicine such as trimeprazine tartrate shortly before bedtime.
- To help reduce the damage that can be caused to the skin by scratching, keep your child's nails clean and cut short. To prevent unintentional scratching at night, your child can wear cotton gloves in bed. Babies can be put into stretch-suits which cover the hands as well as the feet.

Fortunately most children with eczema grow out of it by the age of ten. For more information on eczema, I recommend you read *Eczema and Dermatitis* by Prof Rona MacKie, also in this series.

Seborrheic dermatitis
Unlike childhood eczema above, this condition does not tend to run in families, and it affects a younger age group, appearing most commonly in the first three months of life as a red, scaling eruption on the scalp, face, chest, back and diaper area. The scalp is often covered with hard crusts, popularly called cradle cap. Seborrheic dermatitis does not itch, and its cause is unknown.

Treatment   Your doctor will prescribe cream containing an anti-inflammatory steroid mixed with an antibiotic. This should be applied sparingly, soap avoided and an emulsifying ointment or lotion used for cleaning your child's skin. The skin usually clears completely within a few weeks and in most cases seborrheic dermatitis never returns.

Cradle cap can be removed by applying an over-the-counter ointment containing half strength salicylic acid in soft paraffin for a week. This ointment dissolves the hard crusts of cradle cap. It should be left on the scalp for an hour once a day and then washed off with shampoo.

Diaper rash
Infants' skin is thinner than adults' and is therefore easily damaged by chemicals such as urine. Prolonged skin contact with urine and/or feces encourages the growth of bacteria which break down the urine, producing ammonia, which in turn damages the skin and causes diaper rash. This process is encouraged by the warm, wet environment created by elasticated plastic or rubber underpants. The first sign of diaper rash is redness of the areas closest to the diaper, usually sparing the folds in the groin where the skin is not in contact with the diaper. Without treatment the reddened areas later become infected, producing small ulcers. The skin

may be very tender so that your child cries whenever he or she passes urine.

Treatment   As soon as redness appears, the affected area should be kept clean and dry by changing the diapers frequently and avoiding plastic or rubber underpants except for special occasions. Disposable diapers are preferable to cloth diapers even if your child doesn't have diaper rash, as they are smoother and less irritating to the skin. But if you do use cloth diapers you must wash them thoroughly. A mild detergent is preferable and the washing machine rinse cycle needs to be completed twice. This is to ensure that no particles of solid detergent remain in the cloth diaper and become dissolved when your infant passes urine, thus allowing the detergent to irritate his delicate skin.

   If the rash has become severe you can improve it quickly by not putting diapers on your infant for two or three days and letting him lie on a towel with the affected areas exposed to the air. But this may be difficult to do in practice as extra heating will also be needed for the room.

   An alternative method of treating severe diaper rash at home is to apply compresses soaked in a salt solution several times during the first day. This is not painful. You can make the compresses by soaking cotton gauze in a solution of 1 level teaspoonful (5 ml) of salt to 1 pt ($^1\!/_2$ l) of water.

   In severe cases, when the rash is extensive and perhaps infected and causing your infant distress, your doctor will prescribe an anti-inflammatory steroid cream containing an antibiotic to clear up infection.

   In some cases the rash is also infected with thrush (Candida) – a common fungal infection that may cause white patches to form over affected areas, which, if wiped off, leave a raw surface on the skin. Sometimes, though, thrush will not change the appearance of the original rash, the only symptom being that the rash does not clear after taking the remedial measures already described. If you notice the white patches, or the rash refuses to improve, take your infant to the doctor to confirm the diagnosis. He may prescribe antibiotic nystatin ointment as well as medicine, which should clear up the infection within a week.

   When your infant's skin has recovered, make a habit of generously applying a barrier preparation such as zinc and castor oil ointment or a silicone cream at each diaper change to prevent recurrence of diaper rash. In very mild cases this is the only treatment needed.

'Lick' eczema
Licking the lips or sucking the thumb often causes a reaction in the skin due to saliva. An irritated red area with some scaling spreads from around the mouth and may extend over the whole of each cheek.

   Your doctor may prescribe a mild anti-inflammatory steroid cream which you should apply thinly to the affected patch for a few days until the

1.

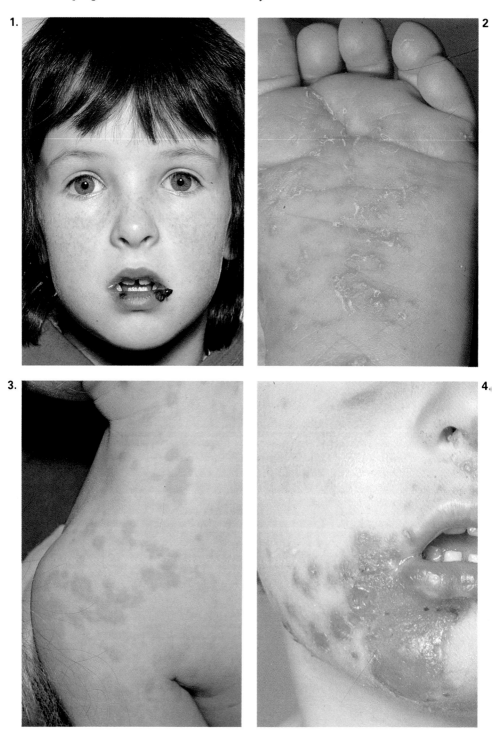

2.

3.

4.

inflammation goes. After that you can apply over-the-counter petroleum jelly or silicone cream to help prevent the chemical effects of saliva from affecting the skin again.

Viral skin problems

Warts

These are small, hard, round swellings on the skin, which are skin coloured. They are particularly common between the ages of six and twelve years, are caused by a virus and are contagious. They are usually found on the soles of the feet, where they are called verrucae, and on the hands but can occur anywhere on the body, and there may be many of them. Verrucae can be painful when they are squashed into the skin of the foot by walking, but warts in other parts of the body do not cause discomfort.

Treatment   Warts often disappear spontaneously and this has given rise to many stories about the success of old folk remedies. What probably happens is that following one of these 'treatments' the wart simply goes away of its own accord, as it would have done had no remedy been tried.

It is best to leave warts alone unless they are painful, are embarrassing for your child, or they appear in groups. When treatment is necessary, you can try simple measures such as covering the wart with a waterproof adhesive plaster and changing it daily. Another treatment which your doctor might recommend is to pare the surface of the wart with an emery board or a pumice stone and apply a prescribed paint of 10–20 per cent podophyllin in tincture of benzoic compound daily for two to six weeks. You should smear petroleum jelly on the healthy skin around the wart to protect it from the irritant effect of the treatment.

If these measures fail, your doctor may freeze away the wart with a liquid nitrogen probe. This procedure is painless, avoids the need for surgical removal with a local anaesthetic and does not produce the painful scar that may result from surgery.

Cold sores

Painful crops of small blisters around the lips and mouth are due to infection with the herpes simplex virus. This ailment is contagious while the blisters are on the skin and may be passed on by kissing. Once the first attack is over, the virus lies dormant in the skin and may set off another attack when your child is not feeling well – usually during a cold. The first attack will be the most severe and may cause ulcers in the mouth,

Opposite: 1. Encrusted cold sores around the mouth. 2. Scabies on the sole of a baby's foot. 3. Urticaria. 4. A fairly severe infection with impetigo.

swelling in the glands in the neck and a raised temperature. The blisters soon burst, forming a crust which lasts for about a week and then peels off leaving no scars. Second and subsequent attacks produce milder symptoms.

Your doctor will not prescribe antibiotics as they only affect bacterial infections. There is as yet no treatment for cold sores in children, so all you can do is wait for the attack to clear up of its own accord.

Molluscum contagiosum

This common and exotically named skin condition is also caused by a virus and can spread rapidly. Pearl-like spots appear, especially on the face and trunk. When you press the spot, a cheesy white material pops out. The spots can disappear of their own accord, or the doctor can remove them painlessly by pricking them with a sharpened orange stick dipped in 10 per cent podophyllin in industrial methylated spirit.

Infestations

Head lice

Epidemics of head lice occur in kindergartens and schools, even where children are well looked after. They may be discovered because your child has an itching scalp or during a routine checkup. On close examination you can see the tiny lice running across the scalp, and their minute white eggs, or nits, sticking to the shafts of the hair. They can also infest the eyelashes, and if your child has scratched his scalp, it may have become infected with impetigo (see page 130). Most parents feel revolted and anxious when their children are infested, but you can be reassured that the head lice are harmless.

Treatment and prevention   If your child has head lice there is no need for him to see the doctor unless his scalp becomes infected. You can use one of the following over-the-counter treatments, all of which should be available from your local pharmacist. One per cent gamma benzene hexachloride in a shampoo base can be applied to the wet hair and rubbed in vigorously to produce a generous lather. Leave the application on for four or five minutes and then rinse the hair thoroughly. One application is enough. As with other antilice shampoos it should not be allowed to touch the eyes.

An alternative is malathion in a 1 per cent cream shampoo which is used in the same way but is effective against certain strains of 'superlice' resistant to other treatment. Also effective against head lice is 0.5 per cent carbaryl lotion.

The common practice of combing out nits with a fine-toothed metal comb is controversial, because once the nits are killed by the shampoo they fall off the hair shafts anyway. They can only stick to them when they are alive. With some preparations, though, some of the lice may only be stunned rather than killed, so combing may be useful.

Children should be persuaded to avoid sharing each other's hats, brushes or combs and encouraged to have their hair washed frequently.

Scabies
This common infestation causes an irritating rash which usually keeps your child awake at night. It is caused by a microscopic mite and is spread by close personal contact, such as cuddling up in bed. It causes red, raised spots, small blisters and black, slightly raised thread-like spots which are the burrows of the mites. The spots may be found on the palms of the hands, the feet (especially the soles), head and neck, and your doctor will confirm the diagnosis by finding one of the mites in a burrow, taking it off the skin and looking at it under the microscope.

Treatment   If you suspect that your child has scabies, he should be seen by the doctor for diagnosis and treatment. He or she will prescribe two applications of 1 per cent gamma benzene hexachloride to all areas of the body, except the face and neck, with twenty-four hours between applications. All people occupying the same accommodation and other close contacts should be treated even if they have no symptoms of scabies. At the end of treatment underwear, pyjamas, sheets and pillow-cases should be washed and ironed. Even after adequate treatment irritation may persist. Go back to the doctor and he will prescribe a 10 per cent crotamiton cream, which usually clears up the problem completely in a week or two.

Other types of skin problem

Urticaria (Hives)
This common, itchy but harmless rash produces red patches and raised white wheals on the skin.

The red patches may have a pale center. Although new spots may continue to develop over a prolonged period, individual spots usually fade within two or three hours, while the larger ones fade after twenty-four to forty-eight hours. At first sight the rash of urticaria is often mistaken for chickenpox (see Chapter 3) or insect bites, but the spots fade faster and do not turn into blisters.

Urticaria may be accompanied by swelling of the lips or eyelids. Very rarely there may be swelling of the larynx, or voice box, producing difficulties in breathing. If your child seems to have trouble with breathing, you should take him immediately to the doctor or your nearest accident and emergency department, where he will be given a shot of epinephrine for quick relief of the swelling.

Causes   Urticaria is an allergic reaction, and is the commonest adverse side-effect of penicillin. It may also be triggered by aspirin and several other drugs, including codeine, atropine and pethidine.

A very large number of foods and food additives have been associated with urticaria, in particular the yellow food dye called tartrazine, and the colouring added to beverages, candies, cookies and cakes. Some pollens can cause the rash in sensitive children.

Treatment   Most attacks are treated with a prescribed antihistamine medicine – either chlorpheniramine or promethazine – which helps to damp down the allergic reaction of the itch. If your child has severe attacks he may need to have anti-inflammatory steroid treatment prescribed by a doctor. If your child has recurrent attacks you should seek the advice of a skin specialist (dermatologist) to try to discover the cause, so that you can try to avoid it in future.

Impetigo
This is a common, highly infectious itchy skin infection caused by bacteria. Thin-roofed lakes of pus form on the face, hands or knees and change rapidly into raw, oozing areas which dry, leaving a golden crust. It may also affect the scalp if your child has been scratching due to infestation with head lice (see previously in this chapter).

You can remove the crusts gently by soaking them with salt compresses (see details in the previous diaper rash section). The raw areas should then be treated with a thin smear of a prescribed antibiotic ointment applied four times daily; your child will also be prescribed antibiotic pills to be taken by mouth. He should stay at home until the rash has cleared – this usually takes about a week with treatment – to avoid infecting people outside the household.

USEFUL ADDRESSES

I hope that in the preceding chapters I have answered most of your questions about childhood ailments and allayed some of your fears. I have already mentioned many of the most likely sources of help for your baby or child: you yourself, your family doctor and other professional specialists. In this appendix are listed the names and addresses of organizations which should be able to help you further.

BRITAIN
British Diabetic Association
10 Queen Anne Street
London W1M 0BD

Coeliac Society of Great Britain and Northern Ireland
PO Box 181
London NW2 2QY

Disabled Living Foundation
346 Kensington High Street
London W14 8NS

Gingerbread
35 Wellington Street
London WC2E 7BN

MENCAP (National Society for Mentally Handicapped Children)
117–123 Golden Lane
London EC1Y 0RT

National Childbirth Trust
9 Queensborough Terrace
London W2 3TB

National Deaf Children's Society
45 Hereford Road
London W2 5AH

National Eczema Society
Tavistock House North
Tavistock Square
London WC1 9SR

Royal National Institute for the Blind
224 Great Portland Street
London W1N 6AA

Royal National Institute for the Deaf
105 Gower Street
London WC1E 6AH

Twins Clubs Association
Porthladd
27 Woodham Park Road
Woodham
Weybridge
Surrey KT15 3ST

UNITED STATES

American Academy of Pediatrics
141 Northwest Point Road
PO Box 927
Elk Grove Village, IL 60007

American Celiac Society
45 Gifford Avenue
Jersey City, NJ 07304

American Organization for the Education of the Hearing Impaired
1537 35th Street, N.W.
Washington, DC 20007

Association for the Care of Children's Health
3615 Wisconsin Avenue
Washington, DC 20016

Association for the Education and Rehabilitation of the Blind and Visually Impaired
2–6 W. Washington Street, Suite 320
Alexandria, VA 22314

Center for Deaf Children
House Ear Institute
256 S. Lake Street
Los Angeles, CA 90057

Children in Hospitals
31 Wilshire Park
Needham, MA 02192

Children's Better Health Institute
Benjamin Franklin Literary and Medical
    Society
PO Box 567
1100 Waterway Boulevard
Indianapolis, IN 46206

National Children's Eye Care Foundation
1101 Connecticut Avenue, N W, Suite 700
Washington, D C 20036

Parents United (Against Sexual Abuse/
    Molestation)
P O Box 952
San Jose, CA 95108

CANADA

Canadian Institute of Child Health
17 York Street
Suite 202
Ottawa
Ontario K1N 5S7

Canadian Medical Association
1867 Alta Vista Drive
Ottawa
Ontario K1G 3Y6

Canadian Pediatric Society
Centre hospitalier universitaire de
    Sherbrooke
Sherbrooke
Quebec J1H 5N4

Canadian Society of Allergy and Clinical
    Immunology
350 Sparks Street
Suite 602
Ottawa
Ontario K1R 7S8

College of Family Physicians of Canada
4000 Leslie Street
Willowdale
Ontario M2K 2R9

Nutrition Society of Canada
School of Food Science
Box 276
MacDonald Campus
McGill University
Ste. Anne de Bellevue
Quebec M5R 2P4

INTERNATIONAL DRUG–NAME EQUIVALENTS

Generic name	UK trade name	Australia trade name	US trade name	Canada trade name
adrenaline epinephrine (US)(C)	Medihaler-Epi (inhaler) Min-i-Jet (injection) see note 1	Medihaler-Epi (inhaler) unbranded preparations	Medihaler-Epi (inhaler) Sus-Phrine (injection) see note 1	Medihaler-Epi (inhaler) Sus-Phrine (injection) see note 1
aspirin ASA (C)	Solprin Levius Paynocil etc see note 1	Aspro Disprin etc see note 1	Bufferin Zorprin etc see note 1	Ancasal Ecotrin etc see note 1
atropine	unbranded preparations see note 1	unbranded preparations see note 1	unbranded preparations see note 1	unbranded preparations
calamine lotion	unbranded preparations	unbranded preparations	unbranded preparations	no information available
carbaryl lotion carbaryl (A)(C) Carabil (US)	Carylderm	not available	not available	not available
chlorpheniramine	Piriton Alunex	Piriton Chloramin etc	Alermine Teldrin etc	Chlorphen etc
codeine	unbranded preparations see note 1	Codate see note 1 unbranded preparations	unbranded preparations see note 1	Paveral (liquid) see note 1
crotamiton cream	Eurax	Eurax	Eurax	Eurax
dicyclomine hydrochloride	Merbentyl	Merbentyl	Bentyl	Bentylol Formulex Protylol Lomine etc
digoxin	Lanoxin	Lanoxin Natigoxin	Lanoxin	Lanoxin Natigoxine
dimethicone cream dimethylpolysiloxane cream (C)	Siopel* Vasogen*	Silcon Dermafilm etc	Covicone Hydropel	Barriere
erythromycin	Erythrocin Erycen Ilosone etc	Erythrocin Eryc Ilocap etc	E-Mycin Ery-Tab Eryc etc	Erythromid E-Mycin Noverythro etc

KEY
* – indicates a product with more than one active ingredient
(C) = Canada; (US) = United States of America; (A) = Australia

Generic name	UK trade name	Australia trade name	US trade name	Canada trade name
gammaglobulin immune globin (C)	Gammabulin Gamma Globulin Kabi	unbranded preparations	Immuglobin Gammar	Gamimune
gammabenzene hexachloride lindane (US)	see note 2 Quellada (lotion) Lorexane (lotion)	Gamene (lotion) Quellada (lotion) etc	Scabene (lotion)	Kwellada GBH
malathion	Prioderm (lotion)	KP24 (lotion)	Prioderm (lotion)	not available
methylcellulose liquid	Cologel	not available as a liquid	Cologel	not available as a liquid
nystatin ointment	Nystatin Multilind	Nilstat Mycostatin	Nilstat Mycostatin	Nilstat Mycostatin
nystatin drops	Nystan Nystatin-Dome	Nilstat Mycostatin	Nilstat Mycostatin	Nilstat Mycostatin
oestrogen estrogen (US)(C)	see note 3	see note 3	see note 3	see note 3
oral electrolyte replacement solution (powder for solution)	Dioralyte Rehidrat	Repalyte	Infalyte Pedialyte	Pedialyte Lytren
paracetamol acetaminophen (US)(C)	Panacol Panasorb see note 1	Paralgin Tymol etc see note 1	Tylenol etc see note 1	Atasol Campain etc see note 1
penicillin	see note 3	see note 3	see note 3	see note 3
pethidine	unbranded preparations Pamergan P100* Pethilorfan*	Pethoid (injection)	Demerol	Demerol Demer-Idine
phenobarbitone	Luminal	see note 1	Solfoton	Gardenal
phenytoin	Epanutin	Dilantin	Dilantin	Dilantin
piperazine citrate	Antepar (syrup) Ascalix (syrup)	not available	Antepar (syrup)	not available
podophyllin in compound tincture of benzoin podophyllin topical solution (US) podophyllin (C)	unbranded preparations	unbranded preparations	unbranded preparations	no information available
promethazine	see promethazine hydrochloride	see promethazine hydrochloride	see promethazine hydrochloride	see promethazine hydrochloride

promethazine hydrochloride	Phenergan	Phenergan Meth-Zine	Phenergan Remsed	Phenergan Histantil
salbutamol albuterol (US)	Ventolin Asmaven Salbulin Cobutolin	Ventolin Respolin	Proventil Ventolin	Ventolin
salicylic acid in soft paraffin salicylic acid in petrolatum (US)(C)	unbranded preparations	unbranded preparations	no information available	no information available
senna	Senokot Senade	Senokot	Senokot	Senokot
silicone	see note 4	see note 4	see note 4	see note 4
sodium cromoglycate cromolyn sodium (US)	Intal (inhaler) Rynacrom (nasal) Opticrom (eyedrops) Nalcrom	Intal (inhaler) Rynacrom (nasal) Opticrom (eyedrops)	Intal (inhaler)	Intal (inhaler) Rynacrom (nasal) Opticrom (eyedrops) Nalcrom
theophylline	Theo-Dur Lasma Theograd Nuelin etc	Theo-Dur Nuelin	Theo-Dur Labid Bronkodyl etc	Theo-Dur Respbid Quibron-T etc
steroid	see note 3	see note 3	see note 3	see note 3
trimeprazine tartrate	Vallergan	Vallergan	Temaril	Panectyl
warfarin	Marevan Warfarin WBP	Coumadin Marevan	Coumadin Panwarfin	Coumadin Warfilone Warnerin
zinc and castor oil ointment	unbranded preparations	no information available	no information available	no information available

KEY
* – indicates a product with more than one active ingredient
(C) = Canada; (US) = United States of America; (A) = Australia

NOTES

1. Drug is present in several multi-ingredient products
2. The official name for gammabenzene hexachloride is now lindane (this note applies to U.K.)
3. The name is a general term, used to describe a group of drugs with similar structure and/or action
4. Silicone is usually understood to be a general term (used with the indefinite article e.g. a silicone), referring to silicon-containing substances. The silicone most often used in creams is dimethicone, hence details of silicone creams are entered under 'dimethicone'.

ACKNOWLEDGMENTS

I wish to thank Dr H. V. L. Finlay and Dr R. J. K. Brown for sharing their extensive clinical experience with me over many years. I am indebted to my wife who has patiently typed and re-typed the manuscript several times.

Bernard Valman 1985

The publishers are grateful to the following individuals and organizations for their help in the preparation of this book:
Medical Illustration Department, Northwick Park Hospital and Clinical Research Centre, Harrow, Middlesex for the photographs on pages 22, 26, 30, 55, 99, 126; Mr D. A. Harrison, Regional Plastic Surgery Centre, Mount Vernon Hospital for the photographs on page 27; the *British Medical Journal* for the chart on page 34; The Health Education Council, London for the photographs on pages 38 and 39; Dr Hillas Smith, Northwick Park Hospital, Harrow, Middlesex for the photograph on page 59; The Department of Medical Photography, Guy's Hospital Medical School for the photographs on pages 97 and 98; Michael Glasspool, FRCS, Orpington Hospital for the photographs on page 103; Professor Ronald Marks, Welsh National Medical School for the photograph (top left) on page 126.
We would also like to thank H. Fereday & Sons Ltd, London N7 for the loan of baby scales and weights shown on page 33; Mothercare, Watford for providing some of the baby and child clothes and props for the studio photographs; The Reject Shop Ltd, Kings Road, London SW1, for additional photographic props.
The photographs were taken by Ray Moller, assisted by Sharon Lowery. Special thanks to the models – Nicholas Haddon (3 years), Emily Marlton (2½ months), Alexandra Metcalf (2 years), Joanna Noel (5 years), Lauren Pain (3 months), Sarah Rees (5 years) – and their parents.
The diagrams were drawn by David Gifford and the international drug tables were compiled by Jennifer Eaton.

INDEX

Page numbers in *italic* refer to the illustrations.